Beyond a Western Bioethics: Voices from the Developing World

Angeles Tan Alora and
Josephine M. Lumitao, Editors

Georgetown University Press / Washington, D.C.

Georgetown University Press, Washington, D.C.
© 2001 by Georgetown University Press. All rights reserved.
Printed in the United States of America
10 9 8 7 6 5 4 3 2 1   2001
This volume is printed on acid-free offset book paper.

Library of Congress Cataloging-in-Publication Data
Beyond a western bioethics : voices from the Developing World / Angeles Tan Alora,
Josephine M. Lumitao, editors.
    p. cm. — (Clinical medical ethics series)
Includes index.
ISBN 0-87840-874-6 (cloth : alk. paper)
    1. Medical ethics—Philippines. 2. Bioethics—Philippines. I. Tan-Alora, Angeles. II.
Lumitao, Josephine M. III. Clinical medical ethics (Washington, D.C.)

R725.5 .B49 2001
174′.2′09599—dc21

                                                            2001023502

Contents

Foreword   v
Leonardo Z. Legaspi

Preface   vii
Edmund D. Pellegrino

From Western to Filipino Bioethics: An Acknowledgment in
Gratitude for Having Been a Colleague in a Marvelous Intellectual and
Moral Journey   ix
H. Tristram Engelhardt, Jr.

Western Bioethics Reconsidered: An Introduction   xi
H. Tristram Engelhardt, Jr.

PART I / FILIPINO BIOETHICS: THE FOUNDATIONS

An Introduction to an Authentically Non-Western Bioethics   3
Angeles Tan Alora and Josephine M. Lumitao

PART II / THE ROLE OF THE FAMILY

The Family and Health Care Practices   23
Letty G. Kuan and Josephine M. Lumitao

The Family versus the Individual: Family Planning   30
Angeles Tan Alora, Danilo Tiong, and Josephine M. Lumitao

Care of the Elderly   40
Victoria Pusung

PART III / THE HEALTH CARE TEAM

Professional Relationships in Health Care   47
Antonio Cabezon, O. P., Edna G. Monzon, and Angelica Francisco

Conscience and Health Care Practices: The Case of the Philippines   52
Letty G. Kuan and Tamerlane Lana, O. P.

Honesty, Loyalty, and Cheating   61
Angeles Tan Alora

Philanthropy and Nepotism   67
Angelica Francisco

PART IV / FACING HARD CHOICES

Ethical Issues in the Pediatric Intensive Care Unit   *75*
Angeles Tan Alora and Mary Jean Villareal-Guno

AIDS in the Developing World: The Case of the Philippines   *81*
Josephine M. Lumitao

Human Organ Transplants   *89*
Danilo C. Tiong

Death and Dying   *94*
Josephine M. Lumitao

PART V / ALLOCATION AND JUSTICE

Allocation of Scarce Resources: Macro-, Meso-, and
Micro-Level Concerns   *103*
Angeles Tan Alora and Josephine M. Lumitao

Ethical Issues in Research   *108*
Angeles Tan Alora

A Tax on Luxury Health Care, Generic Drugs, and a Proposal for a New
Preferential Option for the Poor   *112*
Angeles Tan Alora

The Virtues and Vices of Dumping   *119*
Angeles Tan Alora

APPENDIX / BACKGROUND READINGS

In the Compassion of Jesus: A Pastoral Letter on AIDS   *125*
The Catholic Bishops' Conference of the Philippines

Anti-Abortive Drugs Act of 1995   *130*
Tenth Congress of the Republic of the Philippines

The Patients' Rights Act of 1995   *133*
Tenth Congress of the Republic of the Philippines

Code of Ethics   *141*
Board of Medicine

The Philippines   *151*
Angeles Tan Alora and Josephine M. Lumitao

Glossary   *157*

Contributors   *159*

Index   *161*

Foreword

Leonardo Z. Legaspi, O. P.

The study of bioethics reveals an apparent disparity in application of bioethical principles in the West (the United States and Europe) and in the East (Asia). The secular humanist bioethics that is predominant in the West, which attempts to address complex bioethical issues in a pluralistic society, presents difficulties in a health care setting immersed in a culture deeply rooted in a long religious tradition. Principles of autonomy and justice are differently applied in a culture in which family is a primary value, interdependence an accepted norm, and poverty affects the majority of the population. Hence, the application of Western bioethical principles in the Asian backdrop has been inadequate.

The need to express the reality of this difference was the impetus for this publication. This book is a product of the collective thoughts and reflections of Filipino mentors and students, seriously inclined toward the study of bioethics, who have undergone immersion in poor Filipino communities. Under the guidance of Dr. H. Tristram Engelhardt, Jr., these bioethics enthusiasts gathered in reflective discussions and sharing of their individual insights on bioethical issues in the Philippine context. All of them have been directly responsible for providing health care as physicians, nurses, or pastoral workers to less fortunate Filipinos. They have been involved with the South East Asian Center for Bioethics (SEACB). SEACB was an informal study group in the early 1980s; it evolved into a formal Center after the 1987 visit of the International Federation of Catholic Universities Bioethics Group, headed by Dr. Engelhardt and J. Callus Harvey.

Several articles exploring bioethics in the Asian reality have been published in various journals and other publications. This volume, which is the fruit of the collaborative efforts of promising Filipino bioethicists, is one of the first published books on this subject. It is hoped that this volume will contribute to the growing awareness of Asians and Filipinos, in particular, of the significance of the field of bioethics.

Preface

Bioethics, which is now a worldwide movement, began as an American intellectual and cultural phenomenon. Its philosophical stance has been Western, pragmatic, secular, and strongly influenced by the ideals of liberal democracy. As it has spread in the past decade to the rest of the world, "American" (or "Western") bioethics has encountered some resistance from the older cultures of Europe and Asia. Particularly at issue is the West's insistence on the centrality of individual autonomy, informed consent, and truth-telling and the inadmissibility of religious ideals in public moral discourse.

These transcultural confrontations within the bioethics movement are fueled by the growing worldwide acceptance of the political tenets of liberal democracy. The ensuing transcultural dialogue within bioethics promises to be one of the major challenges to the field's future identity and influence. Certainly, this discussion already is taking place within the United States itself, which now is a culturally diverse nation in which confrontations within bioethics are being played out on a microscale.

This remarkable book, edited and coauthored by two female physicians on the faculty of the University of Santo Tomas in Manila, provides a specific case in point. It shows how, on one hand, bioethics has entered the Filipino medical consciousness and, on the other, how its Western and American character is found wanting in the Filipino context in particular and the developing world in general.

As H. Tristram Engelhardt, Jr., points out in his Introduction, the contributors to this book were introduced to bioethics in the Western world's view in courses in the United States and through visits by American and European bioethicists to the Philippines. They became familiar with the methods of principlism, casuistry, and practical decision making. They were exposed to the culmination in Western bioethics of the post-Enlightenment, anti-metaphysical, anti-religious ethical ethos.

They produced this book after a decade of reflection on what they had learned and what they knew about health care and ethics within Filipino society specifically and the developing world more generally. They faced an enormous intellectual and cultural challenge, which amounted to an encounter with a new sort of imperialism and colonialism—in the intellectual rather than the political realm. The more they applied what they had learned, the more they appreciated the misfit between Western—especially American—ethical values and priorities and their own. Like many Asians and even some Europeans, they especially questioned the virtual absolutization of individual autonomy, which flies in face of the Filipino reliance on the values of community, family, friendship, and church.

The book is filled with concrete examples of the different moral weight that Filipinos place on, for example, telling the truth to patients or families, revealing medical errors, cheating in medical school, or stealing from institutions. In addition, it demonstrates the great moral power of nepotism and the value Filipinos place on loyalty to friends versus loyalty to the law or to institutions. Especially significant is the overwhelming influence of religion in Filipino life—particularly the teachings of the Roman Catholic Church concerning sexuality, abortion, and reproduction.

The editors and contributors tackle thorny issues of allocation of scarce resources in societies where there are genuine scarcities. They show that expressing a "preferential option for the poor" has an entirely different meaning in a developing society in which so many people are poor and high-tech medicine is reserved for the rich and the privileged.

The authors emphasize that many ethical decisions ultimately will be the same in a non-Western ethical culture—but for very different reasons. This similarity holds true for issues of death and dying, organ transplantation, care in the pediatric intensive unit, and care for the elderly, among others.

Drs. Alora and Lumitao have provided an important, interesting, and provocative insight into one sector of the collision between Western and North American versions of bioethics and those pertinent to an Asian Filipino culture. Bioethicists need to learn more about differences in cultural nuance between and within each other's cultures. For American bioethicists, this book will provide a look at how one segment of our own society interprets ethical questions. As medicine becomes a cosmopolitan and global enterprise, different interpretations of what constitutes "bioethics" and how it is practiced will become even more urgent.

Works of this sort also alert us to the reverse side of that coin: How much of bioethics is universal? How much transcends cultural boundaries? What is normative for all humans, and what is not? How are cultural conflicts to be resolved? Is culture self-justifying? Beyond the recognition of differences in cultural ethics lies the troubling fundamental issue of productive dialogue across cultural boundaries. This book and others like it represent the first steps in mapping the topography of what is sure to be an intensive dialogue and dialectic for the next millennium.

Edmund D. Pellegrino

From Western to Filipino Bioethics: An Acknowledgement in Gratitude for Having Been a Colleague in a Marvelous Intellectual and Moral Journey

H. Tristram Engelhardt, Jr.

In the summer of 1986, through the support of the International Federation of Catholic Universities, I began planning a bioethics seminar to be held in Manila with the co-sponsorship of the University of Santo Tomas and the Santo Tomas Hospital. I arrived in the Philippines in March 1987, with colleagues from Argentina, Catalonia, the Kingdom of the Netherlands, Texas, and the United States, including Fr. Francesc Abel, Baruch A. Brody, John Collins Harvey, José Alberto Mainetti, Laurence B. McCullough, Michael A. Rie, and L. B. J. Stuyt. I met people who would become my colleagues on an intellectual journey extending over more than a decade. Following this initial bioethics seminar (March 22–27, 1987), a series of intensive courses was held in Houston (May 10–29, 1987; May 28–June 8, 1990; July 29–August 9, 1991; May 17–28, 1993; and June 11–25, 1997). Other intensive courses were held in Manila (e.g., August 14–18, 1989). Individuals who contributed richly to these undertakings came from Indonesia, India, and Europe, as well as the Philippines and elsewhere. Among these contributors were Angeles Tan Alora, Antonio Autiero, Milagros Banez, Fr. Cornelis Adrianus Maria Bertens, Fr. Antonio Cabezon, Bu Castro, Mark J. Cherry, Rosalinda Concepcion, Lily Coo, Enio Porto Duarte, Felix Estrada, Ruiping Fan, Angelica Francisco, Fr. Fausto Gomez, T. Sintak Gunawan, Rudy Hartanto, Fr. Gerald Healy, Khoe Khing Hien, Robert Imam, Marcelo Irnak, Samsi Jacobalis, Flordeliza de Jesus, A. Sonny Keraf, Lettie Kuan, Philomena Lopez, Jesus Loyola, Jospehine Lumitao, Harry H. B. Mailangkay, A. F. A. Mascarenhas, Ruud H. J. ter Meulen, Edna G. Monzon, Fr. Andres Nowe, Pilar Nunez, Eduardo Pascual, S. Pena, Elizabeth Porras, Mirjam Lusiana Regis Rukmarata, Mark Runge, Nelia Sison Salvacion, Sutanto Sandakusums, F. X. Soediyanto, Rosario J. Sosa, Robert T. Walter, and Fr. Kevin Wm. Wildes. This list is incomplete, but I am very grateful to all who contributed. For example, I must recognize the special inspiration and guidance of the Most Rev. Leonardo Z. Legaspi, O.P., D.D.

As with many such visits by Western scholars, the focus was on bringing the wisdom of the West to the East so that it might learn and embrace our bioethics. Throughout this series of intensive courses in Manila and Houston, Angeles Tan Alora and Josephine Lumitao listened intently and politely but pressed back—holding firm to their own perspective and against the pretensions of the dominant Western secular account of bioethics, which aspires to be the global bioethics. From more than a dozen years of dialogue and reflection, they have produced this volume. I am deeply in debt to my Filipino colleagues for their determination in so creatively holding their own ground and giving this book to their Western would-be instructors for their enlightenment. I am grateful for the support of the International Federation of Catholic Universities, the University of Santo Tomas (Manila, the Philippines), and the Institute of Religion (Houston, Texas), which sustained the endeavors that led to this volume.

Western Bioethics Reconsidered: An Introduction

H. Tristram Engelhardt, Jr.

This is an important work. The authors have succeeded in appreciating bioethics in terms drawn authentically from the developing world. Considering the challenge, Angeles Tan Alora, Josephine M. Lumitao, and their colleagues have done the nearly impossible. They have stepped outside the usual expectations and creatively started anew. They have freed themselves of what some thinkers have termed the Western moral imperialism: the view that liberal cosmopolitan morality born of the western European Enlightenment is the morality that should bind all humans. As a result, the authors have produced a chorus of authentic voices addressing bioethical issues as they arise in the developing world.

The authors accomplished all this despite having received the customary American/western European indoctrination in bioethics, its content, and its methods. Their reeducation began with an open conference at the University of Santo Tomas in Manila, March 22–27, 1987. Westerners explained to the often-astonished Filipino theologians, philosophers, physicians, nurses, and soon-to-be bioethicists how they should understand bioethics in theory and in practice. The bioethics to which they were introduced encompassed the established principlism and casuistry that had become popular in the United States and subsequently in Europe. "Medical ethics" was replaced with "bioethics"— thereby locating the health care professions within a new, post-professional health care ethos. The authors were then invited to the United States to learn first-hand in intensive courses how bioethics is done; they spent considerable periods in Houston, Texas, and Washington, D.C. In the years that followed they also were subjected to several subsequent missionary visits from American and European bioethicists who were sent to the Philippines to introduce the Filipinos to further refinements in bioethical theory and practice. Unique in all of this was a conscious decision from the beginning to present a plurality of Western voices and to involve scholars from Indonesia.

The Filipino bioethicists were then invited to develop a volume addressing health care issues as they present themselves in the developing world.

Initially, the goal was modest. The volume would show how universal bioethics can be applied to the particular circumstances of the Philippines. As they began to write this volume, the authors discovered that Western bioethics and health care policy, which had been offered as the exemplar, nurtured problems of its own—and that it was far from unified. They also realized that many of the difficulties they discovered in Western bioethics were rooted in American and western European post-traditional mores.

The Filipino scholars also confronted the fact that they were not simply being offered morally neutral analytic tools. The very way in which questions were posed in approaching cases and controversies recast the moral agenda. The Filipino scholars found that they were being asked to step into post-traditional, secular, and individualistic Western mores, as well as Western bioethics. They were being led to reconsider their taken-for-granted views regarding the role of religion, the family, and informal arrangements for resolving controversies. Their own moral and cultural commitments as Filipinos were being undermined.

In dialogue among themselves, Indonesian bioethicists, and others, the authors came to appreciate their moral commitments in their own terms. This volume took shape out of an extraordinary sequence of seminars conducted over nearly a decade that examined the bioethical and health care policy choices confronting the developing world. Presumptions of Western bioethics to the contrary notwithstanding, they saw how they could take Filipino morality and its ethics seriously. They also began critically to assess the aspects of Western bioethics that should be embraced, revised, or rejected. They also came to recognize that to live within their own culture and to accept its integrity is to encounter a way of life. From this encounter, they realized that they could offer what no one had yet produced: an authentic vision of the lifeworld of health care and bioethics in the developing world. Out of this experience, the authors articulate what is tantamount to a phenomenology of the medical lifeworld of the Philippines. Like works of art, cultures bring with them fertile insights that are not mathematical theorems, not truths deducible from a sound rational argument. Alora and Lumitao and their colleagues address the Filipino context by laying out its tensions, conflicts, and concerns.

This volume has been more than 10 years in the making. Like good wine, this work has slowly come into its own. As the manuscript was written, revised, and rewritten, it gained a critical perspective of assumptions that frame the field of bioethics in the developing world and in the West. As a result, the reader will find an important contribution to multicultural studies. The authors have succeeded in reconstructing and presenting the moral assumptions that drive Filipino health care and its bioethical reflections. They have not simply provided a geography of values and their connections in the moral life of Filipino patients, nurses, and physicians. They invite the reader into a bioethics that functions quite differently from the discursive moralities of the West. The reader is shown how a morality can avoid explicitly thematizing issues to take Filipino values seriously in their own terms. The reader discovers that moral commitments can be lived without the objectification and thematization that often occurs in the West.

This approach is metacritical. It brings into question the Socratic paradigm of questioning the traditional morality of one's culture. The authors appreciate that the critical eye always distorts and undermines moral insights that cannot be justified as flowing from the very core of reason itself. Enlightenment rationalism, Western individualism, and the anomie of a moral and cultural vacuum are interconnected. As a result, if one challenges moral commitments that cannot be justified in general rational terms, one can evacuate the core from the traditions of a culture. Under the critical eye of the Enlightenment and the expectations it engenders, one's moral assumptions must be justified by sound rational argument or be abandoned. This call for justification inevitably leads to the post-traditional societies of the West. In this process, the richness of the human moral experience is lost—and with it an opportunity to discuss better where the truth lies.

Another limitation surfaced as well. As one assesses the critical attitude of the West, one must recognize that contemporary Western expectations regarding the roles of individuals and families, as well as the ranking of important moral values, cannot themselves be established without begging crucial questions or arguing in a vicious circle. At the foundations of bioethics, the West has no privileged position over the developing world in determining how those value rankings should be made. Moral content comes from true grace, or at least from taken-for-granted assumptions. Discursive reasoning is formal and cannot magically produce canonical content on its own. In addition, much is true that discursive reason cannot understand. The critical attitude—like the surgeon's scalpel—must be used with care and forethought.

This volume contributes to the growing debate about whether bioethics is global or regional. It provides grounds for supporting the regionality of moral insights and for being cautious about claims on behalf of a global bioethics, as well as uniform international regulations in health care policy. The claim is not in favor of a facile relativism. On one hand is a recognition that there can be different moral obligations in different contexts and that the cultural commitments separating many countries are substantial. Different cultures realize different compositions of values in the abundant range of moral concerns that can direct the moral life. On the other hand, a silent criticism of the contemporary, cosmopolitan Western ethos can be detected. The West has lost important moral and social structures—especially those associated with an extended family—that are difficult to recapture. The developing world often is spiritually rich, even when it is financially impoverished.

The authors have produced an extraordinary resource, a foundation on which much can be built. The substantive introductory section constitutes a promising point of departure for considering the possibilities for non-Western bioethics. This portion of the volume surely will have a significant influence on subsequent work. On one hand, it brings into question the dominant Western bioethical paradigm. On the other hand, it suggests ways in which the project of bioethics can be engaged afresh. Subsequent sections of this volume richly illustrate through case studies what a bioethics framed by non-Western assumptions in theory and practice entails. This is not to claim that Western bioethical assumptions are not present and operative in the Philippines. Nor is it a claim that the authors do not address such concerns. Instead, Alora and Lumitao have relocated them in a larger Filipino framework so that Western bioethical conceits can be reexamined for the truth they have. In this work, they are nested in an enveloping moral context that is quite different from the context that is taken for granted in North America and western Europe. These case analyses enable the reader to ask whether and why these Western moral views contribute, distort, or need to be fundamentally reshaped. Here, especially, is where the power of this volume lies. It leads us to think in new modes and creatively about the enterprise of bioethics.

PART I

Filipino Bioethics: The Foundations

An Introduction to an Authentically Non-Western Bioethics

Angeles Tan Alora and Josephine M. Lumitao

The Inadequacy of Western Bioethics for the Developing World

Standard versions of western European and North American clinical medical ethics focus primarily on aspects of the physician-patient relationship. They address issues such as informed consent, rationing, and patient autonomy, as well as physician and patient integrity (see, e.g., McCullough 1994, 1995, 1996). These discussions often fail to note that many of the issues examined under these rubrics are embedded in and function within a particular context constituted by a host of complex local factors. Economically and technologically, for example, moral issues are derivative of a greater industrial and material development than exists in many areas of the world. In developing countries, several worlds of medicine may exist simultaneously; these worlds can be described as affluent worlds versus survival worlds or as first, second, third, and even fourth worlds of health care.

This volume explores the radically different character that bioethics takes in the developing world. It does so by taking as a heuristic bioethics in the Philippines. Although the focus is particular, we believe that the moral is general: The bioethics that developed in the United States in the 1970s and 1980s and purports to provide a global bioethics that is applicable in all countries falls seriously short of this goal. Indeed, this volume explores the challenges for framing a bioethics in the developing world. The Philippines is taken as a case example that captures the developing world at its most interesting juncture. The Philippines is Christian and Islamic; it has been a colony of Spain and the United States but has always remained authentically embedded in its own east Asian traditions.

Within developing countries, society, family, and church assume a moral and religious importance no longer found in the West. In traditional societies, the family takes for granted values such as authority, obligation, honor, and caring. The religious community can straightforwardly assume the meaningfulness of certain beliefs, attitudes, rituals, and symbols. One of the most glaring contrasts between the West and east Asian countries is the character of scientific medicine as it is played out through interactions among patients, physicians, nurses, institutions, communities, and society. Western bioethics reflects moral concerns that, though not necessarily inappropriate for Asian countries, will not adequately capture most moral aspects of their circumstances. Furthermore, contrary to the supposition of some theorists, Western moral analyses, processes, and solutions are not transportable to all bioethical contexts around the world. Consider, for example, Tom Beauchamp's assertion that there are universal rules that all morally serious persons accept. These rules include, among others, the following: tell the truth, respect the privacy of others, protect confidential information, obtain consent before invading another person's body, be loyal to loyal friends, do not cause offense to others (Beauchamp 1997, 26). Although such moral concerns may appear to be *prima facie* significant, they do not capture the spirit of bioethics as it is understood in the Philippines (Andres 1988; Church 1986; Gorospe 1988; Paguio 1991; Miranda 1992). Even rules that do apply in some form must be recast radically to take account of the particular moral context that defines the complex character of Filipino culture. Once recast, such principles often will be dramatically different from their North American and western European counterparts.

The very character of ethics in the West contrasts with ethics in the Philippines not just in terms of the issues and solutions, as well as the context in which each is embedded, but also in the very language and character of moral concern. The focus of Western bioethics is individual; elsewhere it focuses on social units. Western bioethics often is oriented to principles; Filipino bioethics, on the other hand, is not articulated primarily in principles but in lived moral virtues. Whereas Western bioethics is almost always expressed in discursive terms, Filipino bioethics is part of the phenomenological world of living experience. For the West, bioethics is a framework for thought, a conceptual system. For the Philippines it is a way of life, an embodied activity of virtue.

This assertion is not merely a normative claim about the content-rich context of Filipino bioethics. It also is a meta-ethical point, reflecting on the character of moral arguments and claims themselves. It bears on the appropriate framing of cross-cultural ethical debates. The lived phenomenological world of the Philippines cannot be adequately captured in Western discursive moral principles or, indeed, in any particular set of discursive principles. Meta-ethical analysis of the Filipino context not only captures a primarily phenomenological account of how a people conceptualize value, the character of the good life, and moral virtues and obligations; it also can enable Filipinos and others to see the manner in which they grapple with particular normative concerns. For traditional cultures, there is not only a general ethos but also an ethics, and one is bound to be confused and disappointed if one looks for either in the familiar terms of Western ethical analysis (Engelhardt 1996).

In the case of the Philippines, the character of ethical life is more implicit than explicit. It is blurrily defined rather than sharply etched, never fully abstracted from lived reality or defined outside the living context. It is never so theoretically elaborated as to be detached from its *dramatis personae*. Its moral judgments are made not in terms of goodness or correctness alone but also in terms of propriety. Thus, even in dealing with ethics in medicine, the medical circumstance is only one of the many trees in the ethical forest, and medical judgment will not always be the overriding factor.

Although clinical and theoretical bioethicists in the Philippines certainly are concerned with determining the right and achieving the good—to act beneficently, avoid maleficence, be virtuous, and protect the best interests of patients—such appeals must be understood in the context of their moral and religious matrices in the culture. Medicine situates patients and physicians within nests of social expectations, treatment obligations, and understandings of morally licit or illicit medical treatments. Thus, to a large extent the underlying moral content and cultural presuppositions of Filipinos will determine which medical interventions are accepted as morally licit or illicit, as well as which medical policies will underlie what is considered to be effective health care. The cultural ethos is not without influence on discussions occurring in medicine. Indeed, its implicit mode of ethical life ensures that such discussions take on a different valence from Western bioethics. Hence, the Philippines provides an important heuristic for exploring the challenges of framing a bioethics for the developing world.

However accurate this meta-ethical thesis may be, it still does not necessarily imply the moral licitness of any particular normative claim. It does allow us to perceive that this way of life is constituted not only as an ethos but as an ethic. In the Filipino experience, for example, the values expressed in ethics are inextricably fused and woven delicately into each other; they are never expressible as a set of principles to be distinguished rigorously from each other and employed discretely. The resulting texture is one of normative virtues that are not so easily placed into the deontological-teleological taxonomies of the West. It is an ethic whose temper is more consensual than controversial.

One obvious implication is that Filipino health care providers seeking to be authentic bioethicists must listen more self-consciously to their own culture to meaningfully capture its moral vocabulary and speak in terms of its ethical grammar. This process will clarify whether and why they can be its moral friends or its moral strangers.

The bioethical literature is almost entirely dominated by western European and North American scholarship. (For rare exceptions, see Drane 1996 and Hoshino 1997.) Moreover, much of what is written on bioethics in the developing world reflects a dominance of foreign moral paradigms. The literature merely assumes that first-world scholarship, addressing first-world bioethical problems, will apply straightforwardly to developing countries. This volume was conceived to challenge that assumption.

The Complex Facets of Local Religious and Moral Culture

Filipino culture is a complex blend of Eastern and Western influences. This observation does not mean that nothing in the culture is originally Filipino. Such cultural origins are not easily perceivable, however, because Filipino culture is interwoven with many other Eastern cultural characteristics. In addition, the Philippines were subject to Western colonization for many years. Still struggling to overcome the pathos of a colonial mentality, Filipinos also have been forced to contend with the challenge of growing globalization. The global, highly technological, materialistic culture developing in and intruding from the West has a strong influence on a developing country such as the Philippines. Indeed, this phenomenon already is shaping Filipinos' day-to-day lifestyle.

Embedded in this confluence of East and West are religious factors, largely shaped by Roman Catholicism. This religion that was brought to the Philippines by Western missionaries was integrated into Filipino culture without complete abandonment of the native religiosity, which was primarily animistic. Thus, Filipinos have a deep propensity for expressions of popular religion even though they border on the superstitious. This factor accounts for an important ambivalence that is manifested in Filipino behavior with regard to scientific versus miraculous approaches to disease. Not surprisingly, for example, even Filipino Catholics who are strongly rooted in Christian doctrines will not hesitate to express immediate favorable responses to alleged extraordinary phenomena, such as visions and apparitions, even before they receive official recognition from the Church. Also not surprisingly, highly educated Filipinos still seek the unorthodox medical assistance of folk and faith healers, along with the ministrations of the Catholic clergy and professional physicians.

Although specific characteristics typically vary from region to region, between generations, and among social classes, distinctively Filipino patterns of behavior and values can be identified. Several qualifications are in order, however. First, because many of the neighboring Asian cultures share similar beliefs, customs, and values, aspects of the culture that we describe as distinctively Filipino may not be unequivocally and uniquely Filipino. Second, traditionally dominant cultural characteristics are found most distinctively among rural populations, as well as in the lower and middle classes. Urban and upper-class populations have been heavily influenced by the industrialized world's culture, which is *de facto* Western. Although urban and upper-class populations are not the majority, they are sectors of Filipino society that have powerful influence on the lives of others. Hence, the tension between Eastern and the Western cultures is made more manifest. Third, although we point to the fact that Filipinos are predominantly Roman Catholic, highly inculturated non-Catholic Filipinos ought not to be overlooked; for example, there is a small but significant Muslim population. Islam also left a cultural heritage to Filipinos generally, which is essentially integrated into the lifestyle of the indigenous Filipino. Fourth, pointing to such cultural characteristics does not thereby imply that such characteristics are morally appropriate. Such a presupposition would merely justify whatever cultural trends are currently popular, as well as endowing with morally licit status that which is culturally or politically acceptable. Only insofar as cultural characteristics comport with fundamental moral values ought they be judged morally licit. Attention to surrounding cultures, however, does provide essential insights into Filipino patterns of behavior and points to the internal, primarily Christian, morality embedded in their mores. Finally, the Philippines was chosen as a case example precisely because, despite significant external influences, it has remained authentically embedded in its own east Asian traditions.

We focus on representative samples of cultural characteristics that, while functioning as socioanthropological norms, reveal facets of culturally based ethics: the familial community as moral agent; the sociomoral responsibilities of authority; the values of personalism and caring; and the norms and ambiguities of *hiya*, *pakikisama*, *utang na loob*, fatalism, *lusot*, *lakad*, and *lagay*. These norms are particularly relevant to the discussion of what could be considered bioethics in the context of the Philippines.

The Familial Community as Moral Agent

The family is considered to be the social unit of greatest value in the Filipino culture. The family is the core of all social and economic activity. It provides emotional security, economic support, and a deep sense of belonging. Early in childhood, children are taught to be loyal to their family and to know their relatives. Goodwill within the family must be cultivated, and elders respected. Individuals find special pride in being associated with a family of good reputation or shame in being identified with a family of ill repute. Success or failure is measured not vis-à-vis the individual but vis-à-vis the family. Given this strong family ethos, the primary locus of assessment of the good is not the individual but the family. Maintenance of harmony within the family and among peers takes precedence over other concerns for social justice or honesty, which from this perspective appear to be anonymous formal principles that are disengaged from concrete moral community life.

The family ethos reaches into practices such as mutual assistance, group advice, and common decision making. Filipinos can turn to their families and expect from them support in times of need and protection in times of danger. The duty of the family is to protect its members, which often includes not only blood kin but also distant relatives, neighbors, co-workers, peers, and town-mates. Orphans and elderly persons are cared for by the extended family, and unmarried family members generally continue to live in the family home. Important decisions such as the choice of a career or a spouse will involve the entire family, with the head of the family usually considered to be in authority to make the final decision. Even a well-educated and well-employed, but unmarried, young adult is not considered independent or capable of making decisions for himself or herself.

Family interdependence satisfies the need for group belonging and personal identity. This ethos ensures that Filipinos are always confident that there will be people to whom they can turn for physical care and emotional support. Receiving mutual assistance from relatives, godparents, or even co-workers is expected and accepted as normal. Those who provide the assistance accept such activity as their responsibility or duty. As a consequence, Western ideals of individualism and self-reliance have little purchase in the Filipino culture.

The Sociomoral Responsibilities of Authority

Filipinos respect and submit to persons in authority. Character and behavior are shaped under the force of approval of authority figures. This conformity to authority underscores the value placed on maintaining smooth interpersonal relations. It also involves a contrary or paradoxical characteristic: a tendency to preserve a private aspect of one's personality that generally is not revealed to those in authority. Authority figures are shown only public personality traits that are gauged acceptable (see Bulatao 1964, 424–38).

In this context of submission to authority and concern for conformity, respect for parents, elders, and other authorities is strongly emphasized. Psychologically and practically, Filipinos must have the approval of those in authority over them. Plans and projects succeed or fail in direct relation to the authority's support or lack thereof. For example, employees often contribute to a campaign that their employer supports, and community members vote for the candidate that their community leader endorses. If an authority figure disapproves of a plan of action, it will be abandoned outright, or the parties involved will attempt to find a compromise solution. As an unfortunate corollary, persons in authority at times become authoritarian, demanding blind obedience.

Related to the social concern to be respectful of those in authority is an attitude of submissiveness, whereby persons are unwilling to challenge those in authority (Bulatao 1964). Within the family, for example, children are expected to accept reprimands with neither rebuttal nor signs of anger or resentment. Open disagreement with an elder is discouraged. These characteristics translate into a social context in which Filipinos are very respectful, good listeners but reluctant to speak their minds openly. As Bonifacio (1977) describes, Filipinos look to their leaders for support and willingly let those in authority make decisions. Thus, standard Western appeals to the importance of individual liberty often seem out of place in the Philippines.

The Values of Personalism and Caring

Filipino culture is person-oriented: Persons take precedence over abstract, impersonal issues or ideas. For example, a Filipino will feel obliged to violate a governmental obligation if such action can benefit a person to whom he or she has an obligation. This orientation also is reflected in the way in which Filipinos regard reality. Filipinos are said to have an *organic* worldview—an understanding of the world that is quite different from the typical Western architectonic. Concretely, this worldview affects the way in which Filipinos conceptualize reality. Social reality is understood much more subjectively than objectively. Filipinos see and experience the moral world as organized around a network of personal obligations rather than objective moral standards. Therefore, Filipinos begin with personal experience and from these data conceptualize ever deeper insights. Because social reality is accepted as deeply personal, Filipinos have difficulty in distinguishing between philosophical or theoretical discussions and personal arguments. Contrary arguments are taken as attacks against the person. This characteristic at times obstructs the attainment of objective judgments and decisions on important issues.

Within developing countries, abstract philosophical and political issues such as justice or fairness usually are not considered as significant as personal allegiances. In the Philippines, persons in authority tend to recommend, employ, or appoint persons who are related to them, rather than those who might otherwise appear qualified. They are offended if their recommendations are not accepted. Duty, responsibility, and loyalty to persons, especially those in one's family, far outweigh duties or responsibilities to any particular institution. For example, an employee will attend primarily to a friend or mentor, even if doing so will violate company policy.

The person-oriented culture of the Filipinos can best be appreciated in their interpersonal relations, particularly with respect to the aspect of caring. Remnants of *bayanihan* (the communal support and assistance given to a person in need) are still strong, especially in the rural areas of the country. This cultural characteristic also is captured in Filipinos' *pagmamalasakit*, a deep concern for the welfare of the person. Such concern also means that Filipinos make special efforts not to offend or hurt another person's feelings. This attitude takes shape in the manner in which Filipinos communicate with each other. Filipinos are not frank, open people by Western standards. In their desire not to offend others, unpleasant truths, opinions, or requests are stated as pleasantly as possible, and harsh or insulting words are avoided. One aspect of this characteristic is a hesitancy to correct the mistakes of others for fear of insulting them.

Culturally Based Norms and Ambiguities

An adequate picture of moral norms in the developing world would be impossible without careful attention to its particular multi-faceted cultures. In the Philippines, for example, one must consider norms that give rise to a certain amount of ambivalence or ambiguity in Filipino behavior. These cultural traits can be translated into values that by some moral standards appear positive and by other standards are more negative. These phenomena often can be attributed to one of many perceived causes, such as *kahirapan* (i.e., poverty and deprivation—the sad economic plight that Filipinos are struggling to overcome). For example, although the closeness of family ties among Filipinos preserves and strengthens traditional family values that are eroding in the West, extreme economic need has encouraged Filipinos to utilize family connections to obtain access to jobs and positions without regard for qualifications. Nepotism in the government is a frequent occurrence.

Filipino cultural norms and ambiguities are not necessarily alien to the socioanthropological standards of our earlier discussion. In fact, many of these norms are articulations of those culturally based ethical standards. A deeper examination of the norms of *hiya, pakikisama, utang na loob*, fatalism, and the cluster of traits of *lusot, lakad, and lagay* shall be of great help to this study.

HIYA

Conceptually, respect for authority can be captured in numerous Filipino terms, such as *hiya, napahiya, nakakahiya*, and *walanghiya*. *Hiya* describes a painful emotion arising from a relationship with an authority figure or from within a society that inhibits self-assertion in situations perceived as dangerous to one's ego. This emotion is related to the Western concepts of embarrassment, shyness, or timidity, which capture a sense of inadequacy in facing up to something that involves other people whom the individual feels expect too much. Persons who exhibit the virtue of *hiya* do not question authority figures or remark that the authority is acting wrongly.

Napahiya captures a condition that is similar to the Eastern concept of shame, especially among systems of morality that contain separate concepts of shame and guilt. A student who cheats successfully, however, may not feel guilt if he or she is not discovered. For example, if an individual fails to keep his word, he feels ashamed. It indicates a loss of face or self-esteem. Students who fail to provide the correct answer to a question in front of classmates, debtors who are unable to pay their debts on time, or medical students who do not know the expected information will be *napahiya*.

Nakakahiya applies *hiya* to the social context. It pertains to propriety and good manners. For example, visitors will not call during siesta time and subordinates will not telephone a superior; both actions are considered *nakakahiya*. Similarly, *nakakahiya* prevents students who do not understand from asking questions or from airing views that they feel may intimidate the teacher and others. Unfortunately, in so doing, students miss an opportunity to learn or to clarify information.

In contrast, *walanghiya* indicates the absence of the *hiya* inhibition. *Walanghiya* invariably leads to offending others. Subordinates who openly question their superiors are considered *walanghiya*. Although *walanghiya* appears to be negative in the social circle, this type of person who can be aggressive often does well in business. Thus, *hiya* and *walanghiya* both have the potential to undermine an individual's basic interests, given the pervasiveness of authority relations in Filipino society, or to support highly valued relationships and traits.

PAKIKISAMA

Conceptually, the ethos of loyalty, unity, peace, and cooperation demanded by the strong familial community among Filipinos is captured by *pakikisama*. *Pakikisama* is a seeking of harmony with others. At times, individuals may agree to act in ways that they would not otherwise choose to please the group. Personal desires, convictions, and standards are subordinate to those of the group, especially the family. Expressions of *pakikisama* might include taking prolonged coffee breaks with other office workers, doing another student's classwork assignment, or failing to report a sibling's irrational behavior.

A consequence of the depth of these community ties is that intrusions into aspects of life that a Western person would consider to be "private" are frequent. Bonifacio (1977), for example, defines "intrusion" as trying to discover the reasons for an individual action. More literally, the Filipino understanding of intrusion can be translated as *pakikialam* (positive meddling), although the intent is more consistent with *pagmamalasakit* (deep concern). Such intrusion into another person's private affairs does not have an easy, meaningful translation into English. It involves deep concern for the person's well-being and is considered to be a legitimate expectation of social life. With such intrusions, however, there is a concomitant absence of privacy. Filipino culture leaves individuals open to knowledge of each other's social and personal lives. Normal polite conversation may include discussion of intimate personal affairs: how much money a particular person has saved, whom the person is dating, where the person goes, and so forth. Articulating—much less justifying—the force and meaning of a right to privacy is difficult within the traditional Filipino culture.

A side effect of such community bonds is that the group typically finds fault with those who succeed over the group. This individual achievement affects efficiency. Within particular professions, for example, more successful members often are criticized. Their statements at conferences and meetings will be more severely questioned, and minor mistakes will be exaggerated.

UTANG NA LOOB

The depth of the commitment to family and community ties and the ethos of personalism is captured by the phrase *utang na loob*, which expresses a concept of reciprocity or debt of gratitude or honor that imposes corresponding obligations and behavioral expectations. It imposes an obligation on the recipient of a good act or deed to behave generously toward the benefactor for as long as they both live. Within the family, this duty means that children are expected to provide for their parents in old age because the children owe not merely life to their parents but also a lifetime of education. Unlike North America and much of western Europe, where family unity and family commitments often are weak and ineffective, in the Philippines the family bond remains intact and sustains effective moral obligations for support and care, including health care. *Utang na loob* also extends to elder brothers and sisters who have helped in the rearing and education of younger siblings. A child who does not pay this debt of gratitude is said to be *walang utang na loob*, an ingrate. Individuals who are known to be *walang utang na loob* risk being avoided or being a target of reprisal and at times forfeit the security of their social group.

Outside the family, the *utang na loob* relationship is established after a gift is given, either voluntarily or after a request. Acceptance of the gift indicates the creation of a duty on the part of the receiver to reciprocate through some future demand made by the giver. Otherwise, the gift is rejected. Forms of repayment need not be specified. Indebtedness may alternate between the giver and receiver until complete reciprocity of mutual support has been achieved and both become equally indebted and complementary *utang na loob* partners.

When the *utang na loob* relationship involves a superordinate (i.e., a person from a higher social status), repayment is never considered complete.

Utang na loob often affects the distribution of goods, resources, and burdens within the social life of Filipinos. Positions and jobs frequently are allocated according to indebtedness. Likewise, some people exempt others from burdensome responsibilities as a show of gratitude for favors done in the past. In short, instances of a mutual show of gratitude fail Western notions of egalitarianism. Issues of fairness and justice may never become relevant, let alone decisive.

FATALISM AND DEEP RELIGIOSITY

Fatalism—which for American ethicists constitutes a shrinking away from responsibility—is captured by the *bahala na* attitude among Filipinos. There is a heterogeneous cluster of concepts identified as *bahala na,* however. It includes a fatalistic resignation. It expresses a feeling of helplessness in the face of a difficult situation, a withdrawal from personal engagement, or a shrinking away from responsibility for events. The concept also includes an attitude of bravado in the face of existing odds. An acceptance of necessary risk prompts the Filipino to do what must be done even if the prospect of success appears bleak. Filipinos generally are concerned, but not oversolicitous, about events that they are unable to control. Acceptance of the possibility of misfortune is merely a matter of faith. This faith is the richer meaning of what also may be considered a type of fatalism that is particularly Filipino: *Bahala na* at times indicates a deep religious trust in God.

In a survey reported by F. E. Miranda (1990), 61 percent of the respondents ranked trust in God as the most important value for child-rearing. This result was the same across all income groups and for urban and rural respondents. Trust in God pervades many facets of Filipino life. Roman Catholicism and other Christian denominations of faith are instrumental in deepening this attitude. About 80 percent to 85 percent of Filipinos are Catholic. There also are a significant number of Muslims in the Mindanao area, and many non-Catholic Christians in the archipelago. Filipinos are deeply religious. Few would avow agnosticism or atheism. Their fervent religious spirit is vividly evident in attendance at religious ceremonies, joining devotional processions, visiting shrines, and fondness for religious articles such as rosaries and images of Sto. Niño (the Child Jesus), the Sacred Heart, and Mary. Yet although this trusting attitude is always present, at times the focus on rituals and other external forms of worship takes precedence over the inner living of the faith. Expressions of faith may not even be internalized or externalized in other concrete, practical dimensions of Filipinos' lives. Filipinos can be devoted Sunday Mass-goers while living a morally contradictory life the remainder of the week.

LUSOT, LAKAD, AND LAGAY

Lusot, lakad, and *lagay* represent important, although perhaps somewhat less flattering, aspects of Filipino culture. *Lusot* literally means to escape from something via a loophole or through an opening. This concept points to a concern with escaping from an undesirable, unpleasant, or altogether difficult situation as swiftly and painlessly as possible. It often implies avoiding responsibility or escaping from a difficult situation with cunning. Speeding without getting caught by the police or being paid by an employer without doing work are examples of *lusot.*

Lagay is a small gift or amount of money that is used to avoid delay in the release of goods or to obtain access to a scarce commodity, including health care. Filipinos often refer to this money as coffee money, *pang kape,* or *pangmerienda.* On the other hand, *lakad* is an attempt to smooth out such difficulties by using a network of personal connections. When bureaucracy and red tape hinder the accomplishment of a task, one might approach a relative or friend in the office to assist. Before or after the encounter, a bit of *lagay* will smooth the process. For many Filipinos, *lusot, lakad,* and *lagay* are not considered wrong or blameworthy. Faced with the abstract interference of the law and a recalcitrant bureaucracy, *lusot, lakad,* and *lagay* are practical, personal methods of resolving conflicts while maintaining ethically important personal relationships.

Bioethics and the Developing World's Medical Context

Bioethics in the developing world is shaped and directed by its culture as well as by its understanding of fundamental religious values. Clinical encounters, medical education, and research—as well as the very nature of the health care debate in the Philippines—take place within this moral setting, framed by religious values and particular metaphysical understandings such as the existence of God, saints, and malign spirits. In addition to the cultural, moral, and metaphysical commitments that shape the biomedical context of the Philippines, this volume closely examines particular bioethical concerns. These issues include clinical decision making with regard to health care delivery, especially as it deals with death and dying; family planning; human experimentation; and other biomedical issues that can be fully expressed only in Filipino moral categories.

Consider, for example, the distinctively Filipino way of caring for persons who are sick and dying. The close family ethos affects the applicability of the primarily Western concept of autonomy. With the onset of illness, the sick person becomes a family member in need who brings into the clinical setting his or her social support network. The entire family participates in the care of the patient. A family member typically accompanies a patient when he consults his physician or is hospitalized. This family member acts as aide, interpreter, and advisor; helps move the patient around; provides the patient's medical history; and participates in and even exempts the patient from any decision making. An ill family member is admonished not to worry about anything, to focus on resting and becoming healthy again. Business and home matters are taken care of by other family members, who protect the patient from stress and psychological harm. Assured that others will take care of and support him or her, the sick family member accepts a role of dependency and passive tolerance, leaning on the family as a direct source of strength and support.

In contrast to Western notions of free and informed consent or patient confidentiality, the Filipino health care setting focuses on the family and those in authority over the patient. The concept of patient usually refers to the person in need of health care, together with his or her family (i.e., parents and elder relatives). Autonomous, independent patients are the exception. Truth telling is accorded not to the patient but to his or her family. Health care decisions are family decisions. Spouse, parents, and all competent family members participate in weighing alternatives whose resulting benefits and burdens they must share. In the spirit of harmony and in accordance with respect for those in authority, all family members are expected to concur if the head of the family chooses a treatment alternative. Consent forms for surgery or aggressive measures are signed by the senior family member, who often is the most prosperous family member. As with other cultures on the Pacific rim, Filipinos understand the importance of the family acting as a unit to care for its members (see, e.g., Hoshino 1997).

Clearly, the Western moral principles of autonomy, beneficence, nonmaleficence, and justice contrast with Filipino moral concerns; from the Filipino perspective, the former are starkly individualistic, atomistic, and marked by a degree of anomie. Filipino bioethics as a lived ethic does not focus on individual consent to health care, individual confidentiality, or individually articulated concerns with beneficence, caring, and truth-telling. The focus is on family—a social reality that sustains a communal morality. These attitudes are unmistakable deviations from Western secular moral concerns with truthtelling, confidentiality, and informed consent. Such concerns are considered less important than compassionate patient management. In this regard, Filipino families and patients have expectations that are similar to members of certain subpopulations in the West that have maintained similarly robust family bonds (e.g., Indians and Italians).

The choice of a physician and the physician's acceptance of the role of health care provider for a specific patient are affected by personalism, caring, *hiya*, *pakikisama*, and *utang na loob*. Often a particular physician is chosen because he or she is known to the family or has treated a family member before, regardless of whether the specific disorder is part of the physician's expertise. Similarly, the physician agrees to care for the patient because of *hiya* or *pakikisama*. The physician will not want to shame the family by refusing to heed their request and will want to retain a smooth interpersonal relationship.

With *bahala na*, patients agree to be operated on and then leave the problem to God and the surgeon. Decision making can be slow because everything is understood to be controlled by God or fate. The family may wish to wait for signs from God. Moreover, even when health care costs become prohibitive, the family might not withdraw treatment. Indeed, Filipino families commonly instruct the health care provider to do everything possible and then pray for a miracle for the patient while hoping that the financial problem will resolve itself. Because death and dying are negatively valued in Filipino culture, they are rarely spoken of directly. Truth is communicated through euphemisms or indirect behavioral clues. Once death is accepted as inevitable, however, it is somewhat more easy to withdraw life support. After the initial reaction of denial, most Filipinos accept as fate or God's will the truth that they are dying. Suggestions to withdraw life support measures are then much easier to accept.

Physicians often are made to bear the burden of timely declarations regarding the inappropriateness of further treatment, which is a manifestation of their authority position. They take care, however, to ensure that such pronouncements are never misunderstood as entailing patient abandonment. Physicians will continue to care for their patients by listening, spending time with them, and sometimes even praying with and for them. North American physicians who often claim to be bound by commitments of value neutrality probably would find such an active religious role uncomfortable.

The ultimate commitments of the Filipino family help make dying easier and more meaningful by ensuring supportive care. Most Filipinos who are terminally ill choose to leave the hospital to be among the people they love in familiar surroundings when they die. If a patient is unable to return home, a private room where family members can stay is much preferred over a busy intensive-care unit (ICU). The love and support of the family provide the best environment for the Filipino to face the reality and finality of death. It also assists families in coping with the dying process.

Deep connections to family and religious values affect all attempts at what Western cultures would consider rational family planning. Children are accepted as gifts of God who assure continuance of the family name, economic security in old age, and public testimony of the moral and pious lives of the parents. With *bahala na*, the Filipino couple will accept as many children as God sees fit to grace them with and then trust that God will provide for their care. Such an attitude is not conducive to a couple's goal of limiting the number of children. It is conducive, however, to protecting children from harm. Parents work to provide education, health care, and an appropriate living environment for their children. These overarching concerns weigh heavily on the family. In desperate circumstances, a senior family member may even attempt to sell a kidney to raise capital to support his or her family. Such a sacrifice indicates the strength of the love within a family.

A primary concern in the Filipino health care context is the potential abuse of authority. In the physician-patient relationship, physicians are considered to be in authority because of their expertise in medicine and the fact that they usually are from the upper economic and social class. As authorities, physicians are to be respected and obeyed. They hold the keys to life and death and are considered to be second only to God in healing power. Given this circumstance, patients tend to be submissive and inhibited in their relations with physicians and in their compliance with their doctors' orders, often simply deferring to the doctor's decisions. Refusing a particular diagnostic test, treatment regimen, or proposed participation in a research project would be unthinkable for a Filipino patient. *Hiya* prevents patients from asking for explanations, even if they do not understand. In general, in case of disagreement or dissatisfaction the Filipino would rather seek the care of another physician.

A physician may not take the time or effort to obtain what Western bioethicists would consider morally appropriate informed consent. The paternalistic context of Filipino medicine does not regard consent as a necessary aspect of the physician-patient relationship. Physicians are understood to be in authority over the patient's medical care and authorities concerning the patient's best medical interests. The physician's judgment is to be respected because the physician possesses a level of knowledge that creates social authority. At times this paternalism and authority may even be expressed verbally in statements such as, "If you have no confidence in my judgment, why did you come to see me?" or, "You came to see me because you know that I know what is best." One should not conclude that the Filipino patient regards physicians as autocratic or domineering figures. The point is that physicians are expected to be benevolent parental figures who will care for the best interests of their patients.

Within the health care team, the consultant physician is the highest authority. The authority hierarchy moves downward through the resident, intern, nurse, and therapist. During hospital rounds it is highly exceptional for a resident to question a consultant or for an intern to openly disagree with a resident, even when confronted with apparently inappropriate medical choices.

In the provision of health care, a health care provider may assist in a procedure that he or she otherwise would not have performed. A colleague also may not call attention to a misdeed or error by a colleague. As a consequence, there would be a felt moral obligation not to call a colleague's attention to an act of medical negligence. Such behavior is captured under the rubric of *pakikisama*.

Lusot, lakad, and *lagay* are engaged in obtaining health care, in admission to education and training programs, in appointments to faculty and administrative positions, and in the awarding of research grants. Because of personalism, health care providers recognize their duties and responsibilities to particular patients and do what is in their best interest. Unless the physician also is an administrator, however, he or she seldom recognizes strong responsibilities to the hospital or institution in which he or she works. In times of conflict, the physician often behaves as a patient advocate, fighting for appropriate and adequate medical care. This attitude may be best for the individual patient, but it may not assist in the efficient use of scarce resources.

Utang na loob often dramatically affects the allocation of scarce health care resources. If the only bed in an ICU is reserved for a patient to whom the physician or administrators are indebted, this situation will prevent others in greater need of care from receiving treatment. Residency positions sometimes are allocated to the son of an *utang na loob* partner. Many school and hospital policies even include provisions that officially give priority status to such relationships. Again, the Philippines offers a heuristic of the ways in which social webs are inescapable and essential aspects of life in much of the developing world.

In short, Filipino bioethics cannot be adequately articulated in impersonal or abstract principles. It must be understood as a way of life. One must live it to understand it. For many Filipinos, a bioethics that can fully be captured in principles will suffer from anomie, weakness and decrepitude of family structures, and the impersonal character of secular North American bioethics. Filipinos usually do not meet as moral strangers. They meet within a rich and living social fabric that entails obligations of care, support, and concern that generally do not exist in North American culture. Because patients and physicians generally are not morally opaque to each other, there is a shift in the burden of proof. Rather than needing to establish that one is a moral friend, as in the North American moral context, in the Philippines one must establish that one is in fact a moral stranger. The moral concerns of the other do not appear as *prima facie* opaque, as alien facts to be discovered, but as transparent, congenial, and already understood. Indeed, the other is never initially anticipated as radically other but as someone like oneself, with whom one shares beliefs, hopes, expectations, and a content-full common understanding of the good life and the nature of appropriate medical practices. The burden of proof is shifted in favor of persons in authority, in favor of paternalism, community, personal relationships, and personal obligations.

Concerns with health care delivery, education, and research must be placed within the particular cultural, religious, and metaphysical context of particular developing countries. Such concerns, however, set much of the developing world in direct contrast with the world of Western bioethics. Only if such regional characteristics are taken seriously will bioethics be truly applicable to the Filipino context, content, and circumstances. The manner in which appeals to moral virtue, rights, and consequences can be understood and analyzed, to lay out the ethical context of medicine, must be understood within the lived phenomenology of the Filipino context.

The intent of this volume—through its essays, case studies, and overview of the Filipino situation—is to address the fundamental challenges of framing a bioethics in the developing world. It is to take the moral perspective of the Philippines—indeed, of the developing world—seriously. Only then will we be able to have open, honest discussions about the problems facing health care in the Philippines as Filipinos themselves experience these problems. Only then will we will able to have honest bioethical discussions with western European and American bioethicists. We must first acknowledge our differences.

References

Andres, T. Q. 1988. *Understanding Filipino Values*. Quezon City, The Philippines: New Day Publisher.

Beauchamp, T. 1997. Comparative studies: Japan and America. In *Japanese and Western Bioethics*, edited by K. Hoshino. Dordrecht, The Netherlands: Kluwer Academic Publishers, 25–48.

Bonifacio, M. F. 1977. An explanation into some dominant features of Filipino social behavior. *Philippine Journal of Psychology* 10: 29–36.

Bulatao, J., S.J. 1964. Hiya. *Philosophical Studies* 12: 424–38.

Church, A. T. 1986. *Filipino Personality: A Review of Research and Writings*. Manila: De La Salle University Press.

Drane, J. 1996. Bioethical perspectives from Ibero-America. *Journal of Medicine and Philosophy* 21, no. 6: 557–679.

Engelhardt, H. T., Jr. 1996. *The Foundations of Bioethics*, 2nd edition. New York: Oxford University Press.

Gorospe, W. R. 1988. *Filipino Values Revisited*. Quezon City: National Bookstore, Inc.

Hoshino, K. (ed.). 1997. *Japanese and Western Bioethics: Studies in Moral Diversity*. Dordrecht, The Netherlands: Kluwer Academic Publishers.

McCullough, L. 1994. Issues in clinical ethics. *Journal of Medicine and Philosophy* 19: no. 1: 1–19.

———. 1995. Issues in clinical ethics. *Journal of Medicine and Philosophy* 20, no. 1: 1–105.

———. 1996. Issues in clinical ethics. *Journal of Medicine and Philosophy* 21, no. 1: 1–109.

Miranda, D. M.. 1992. *Buting Pinoy*. Manila: Divine Word Publications.

Miranda, F. E. 1990. *Filipino Values and Our Christian Faith*. Manila: OMF Lit. Inc.

Paguio, W. C. 1991. *Filipino Cultural Values*. Manila: St. Paul Publications.

PART II

The Role of the Family

The Family and Health Care Practices

Letty G. Kuan and Josephine M. Lumitao

The Family Constellation

In developing countries, the family assumes a moral importance it no longer has in the West. Authority, community, personalism, and caring—combined with a particular constellation of family dynamics—define lived Filipino culture; they shape the character of health care and dramatically recast issues such as informed consent, patient confidentiality, and treatment compliance (Andres 1985). The family—typically composed of parents, children, and extended relations—is the basic social unit of the Philippines. The Filipino family is quite extensive. Relatives beyond the third degree are recognized, and relationships are strongly established. Furthermore, Filipino kinship is bilateral: Any member of the extended clan will claim an equal relationship with the kindred of his or her father and mother. As Mendez et al. (1984) documented, this bilateral reckoning of relationships encompasses a large group of individuals with overlapping roles, as well as rights and obligations.

Many Filipino cultural characteristics are experienced, expressed, and made relevant in the context of the family. The family is a social support system that can always be relied on to protect and provide security for its members. As the anchor of the Filipino social system, the family influences bureaucratic practices, professional decision making, and customary action in health care. According to Mendez et al., in the proper perspective the family can even hasten the development and patterning of new values that support national unity. Almost all social organizations and community activities offer evidence that the family is central in Filipino society.

Most decision making takes place within the family structure. When decisions must be made, family members discuss the matter and together come to a conclusion. This influence is evident in the choice of careers, marriage partners, occupations, religion, and health care practices. Children and parents most often practice the same religion, which is advantageous because the shared practice facilitates unity and closeness among family members. Family interests take precedence over those of the individual members. Mendez et al. (1984), for example, opine that because of family primacy, the honor of the family usually is at stake when an individual family member errs. Similarly, whenever a family member is successful in a profession—such as when one passes the legal bar, a state board examination, or wins an election—the family usually receives more accolades than the individual.

The family has a significant influence on the choice of interventions during health care emergencies and times of illness, as suggested by the results of a study done in 1975 (Kuan 1976). Two hundred respondents living in Project 1 of Quezon City who came from the three-island grouping of Luzon, Visayas, and Mindanao were queried about their concepts of health and corresponding health care interventions in times of emergency and illness. The study found that 94 percent of the respondents were influenced by their families (especially their parents) in making decisions about appropriate care. Respondents who had been living with their parents and grandparents during the first 15 years of their lives tended to approach health care in the same way as their parents. Regardless of the respondents' educational level, during emergencies and in times of illness they consulted their parents and followed their parents' advice. For example, when parents suggested consulting an herb healer, the individual did not hesitate to do so in spite of his or her degrees or college diploma.

Implications of the Family Structure

The closely knit structure of the Filipino family renders unacceptable Western principles such as autonomy, informed consent, and confidentiality. When a family member falls ill, he or she is considered to be in need of protection from the harmful effects of knowing the diagnosis, as well as the stress of decision making. Family members automatically take the role of patient advocate, even requesting that the patient not be told the diagnosis. The dominant authority figure (the mother or father) together with older extended relatives take it upon themselves to talk with the physician and decide among treatment options. Patients generally are protected from such stressful information and difficult choices. Only when the patient specifically asks about the diagnosis may his or her claim to a right to know be recognized. Granting this right, however, depends on the family's perception of the patient's claim, which depends on the patient's status in the family (e.g., age and educational attainment), as well as the patient's perceived strength and capacity to handle the information. At times, the wishes of an individual patient will be overruled if the family decides otherwise.

Patients, for their part, do not hold a grudge or complain to physicians for divulging information to their families. Indeed, Filipinos accept the fact that the family will know about the sick family member's disease and overall prognosis. The extra chair in the doctor's clinic is for the relative who accompanies the patient during consultations. In the Philippines, nobody considers it unethical for relatives to be present when the diagnosis is divulged. During a consultation, the physician sometimes talks to the relatives first, especially if the relative is older, as if the patient were not present at all. Autonomy and confidentiality—values or principles that are recognized and protected in Western culture—are nonexistent, or at least marginalized, in Philippine health care.

There also are notable differences in the way informed consent is obtained in the Philippines. A sense of harmony concerning relationships is valued in this culture. Sickness is "unpleasant news" that disrupts such harmony. Within the paternalistic, benevolent context of Filipino health care, information is couched in euphemisms or terms acceptable to the culture (for example, *bukol* or "mass" instead of cancer, "weak lungs" instead of pulmonary tuberculosis). The other exceptional difference is that usually the family, not the patient, asks for and receives information. Moreover, the family gives consent regarding treatment options. Filipinos presume that the best interests of an individual patient will be best protected by a decision made by the family. Individual patient autonomy is an alien concept within Philippine health care. Insisting on such autonomy would suggest a problematic anomie: existence outside of the context of a functioning family.

The family also determines the physician who will be consulted in times of sickness. If a family member becomes ill, the family consults other relatives first and then seeks a physician recommended by the relatives. Such referral is based less on whether the particular physician is a specialist in the field of the patient's disease than on the fact that the relatives know the physician. This phenomenon is an expression of the cultural value of personalism. Yet even in such cases, the patient would place all trust in the doctor's capacities, whether the physician manages the patient himself or herself, albeit inadequately, or refers the patient to a colleague who is a specialist. This situation offers potential ground for abuse from mismanagement of the patient because of inadequate skill or from double professional fees. Yet in the Philippines, this approach is considered a risk worth taking and a cost worth paying.

Family members also play a substantial role in determining whether a patient will comply with medical advice. Because family practices are strongly ingrained in the minds of young people, they have a tendency to do what the family recommends rather than to heed the advice of the health practitioner. For example, if a physician restricts a patient's salt intake because of hypertension but the patient's family believes that salt is a necessary element in daily food intake, the patient would be likely to continue to consume salt and disregard the doctor's advice. Relatives inquiring about a family member's prescription medication may then persuade the patient to stop taking all medications, before consulting with the relative's physician. Furthermore, physicians usually take care of patients who belong to the same family. For example, an obstetrician who takes care of one pregnant patient will then be endorsed by that patient to her sisters, cousins, and other extended family and friends. The first patient in the family may even take the time to accompany the referred patient to her physician.

The family also functions as the primary, and often only, support system in times of sickness. Just as the family asks about the diagnosis and decides on treatment options, it also takes upon itself the role of being a social support network during the healing process. Immediate members of the family, as well as extended relatives, also contribute in whatever way they can to relieve the financial burden incurred by the patient. They also take turns visiting the patient in the hospital. In the case of a seriously ill or dying patient, this concern is even more evident because the visiting relatives bring along their religious friends.

All of these actions are undertaken in a spirit of loving concern to protect the patient from the stress that his or her sickness brings. The patient ought to concentrate solely on getting well. When the patient is the dominant authority figure, all of the sons and daughters—no matter how far away they live—understand their responsibility to come home and do their share in taking care of their sick parent. This behavior is an expression of *utang na loob* at its highest level because children grow up with a deeply ingrained sense that they owe their lives and whole being primarily to God, and only secondarily to their parents.

Filipino patients have a family to lean on for support, nurturing, and strength in times of illness and death. The all-encompassing character of the family and the authority it possesses may appear out of place, if not pernicious, to physicians, nurses, and others from post-traditional societies. They will have no perspective from which to anticipate how different a traditional culture's expectations are.

Illustrative Cases

CASE 1: Diego, a 76-year-old married male, was rushed to the hospital because of severe abdominal pain. He was diagnosed with a hepatocellular malignancy. At the hospital, Diego was accompanied by his wife, niece, and son, who brought him for his various diagnostic exams. The hospital chaplain visited Diego at the request of a relative. Diego's son was informed by the physician of his father's diagnosis. The son then asked that the diagnosis be revealed to Diego only if Diego explicitly asked but that the prognosis be withheld regardless of Diego's questions. Upon learning of his diagnosis, Diego asked to be brought home.

Four of Diego's married children who were residing abroad immediately traveled home to take care of their father. Close members of the family, as well as more distant relatives from the province, came to visit. Their parish priest saw Diego often, anointing him and bringing communion. Diego died peacefully at home, surrounded by his loving family, grandchildren, and extended relatives.

ANALYSIS: This case illustrates the ways in which Filipino families reach out in love to care for their family members. Diego was the dominant authority figure. His illness divested him of his authority, however, and reduced him to the status of a sick family member in need. The fact that Diego's son still recognized his status is illustrated, however, by the way in which he acknowledged Diego's right to know his diagnosis. The son's request to withhold the prognosis can be understood as a concern to shield his father from the harmful effects of a bleak prognosis.

Another issue that this case illustrates is the social support role played by the family for a sick and dying family member, especially a parent. Although the four children who lived abroad lived in thoroughly secular environments, they did not lose their sense of family commitment. Thus, as an expression of compassion and family connectedness, they left their jobs to return home to care for their dying father. Sickness and death may be difficult to face, but the Filipino family support system will do its best to ease this trying time, rendering such suffering bearable.

CASE 2: Basilia, a 75-year-old active diabetic female, requires amputation of her gangrenous right leg. Basilia's daughter, knowing that her mother will refuse surgery, gives consent, instructing the surgeon not to inform her mother.

ANALYSIS: This case illustrates a decision that is entirely unacceptable in Western culture, morality, and bioethics: the family (in this case the daughter) providing consent for the mother's leg to be amputated without the patient's prior knowledge or consent. Although the patient is an authority figure, her sickness places her in the category of a sick family member who needs to be protected from her refusal of treatment. The family entirely disregards the patient's wishes. It acts as a court would to acknowledge a guardian. All of this behavior occurs within the fabric of an intact traditional morality.

Basilia, for her part, may go through a gamut of emotions after the surgery, beginning with anger. This anger will later subside to relief, with a mixture of fatalism and gratitude. After all, this is what being part of a family entails. Along with these emotions will emerge the realization that her daughter decided on this course of action out of concern for her mother's well-being and safety. In the end, Basilia will accept the family's decision.

Western medical ethical principles may consider this situation highly unethical. From the Filipino family's perspective, however, the choice by the daughter is morally obligatory. In the role of caring for a sick family member, such action by a family member—even to the point of disregarding the individual's consent—is understandable and acceptable. The only issue is to identify the family member who is in authority, a matter that usually is clearly dictated by traditional morality.

CASE 3: Mr. Chonco, a 52-year-old business executive, is partially paralyzed following a stroke. His family calls for Dr. Duran, an orthopedic surgeon who is a family friend, to take care of Mr. Chonco. A private nurse notices that Mr. Chonco's condition is worsening. Against her better judgment, she musters enough courage to suggest that Dr. Duran refer Mr. Chonco to a neurologist who will be able to provide more specialized care. At this suggestion, Dr. Duran becomes angry and insulted, insisting that he is the only physician the family trusts.

ANALYSIS: This case illustrates the role of the family in deciding on the physician who will take care of the patient, based on "personalism" rather than "expertise." The nurse (an unusually outspoken and courageous nurse from the Filipino point of view because the culture does not encourage confrontation with authority figures) plays patient advocate and suggests a referral. Dr. Duran (who is in the position of authority, even though he may not be the best medical authority)[1] considers the suggestion a personal affront rather than an effort to improve Mr. Chonco's care. The almost reverential trust of the family in a personally known physician is rich ground for abuse and patient mismanagement, as well as a source of special care and attention. In traditional Filipino culture, physicians such as Dr. Duran should accept their limitations and advise the family that Mr. Chonco should be referred to a neurologist. He also should reassure the family, however, that he will co-manage Mr. Chonco's treatment to allay the family's fears and anxieties about the intrusion of an unknown physician.

Conclusion

Within the developing world, the family provides an extended social network for individuals. The family is the basic unit of Filipino society; it plays a central role in all aspects of an individual's life.

The family influences health care in several important ways. First, closely knit family and friend relationships make maintaining Western concerns for confidentiality difficult or even impossible. Moreover, such standards of confidentiality are regarded as morally inappropriate—as attitudes that distance individuals from their families. Individual autonomy gives way to joint family decision making in obtaining informed consent.

Second, because individuals tend to rely heavily on their families, a patient may follow his or her family's advice instead of following the physician's orders; noncompliance with treatment regimens often results. Physicians must recognize this pattern to secure appropriate compliance.

Third, the family may consider personal relationships to be the most important factor in choosing a physician, rather than the physician's expertise and skill. Likewise, a physician may care for a patient because of his or her relationship with the family, not because the physician is competent to provide appropriate care for the patient. Even after a patient's condition worsens or fails to improve, the family may be reluctant to find another physician. The physician likewise may not suggest another doctor to take his or her place. Although this situation may appear to reflect a lack of professionalism, it captures the close relationships among family members and friends that reach out to envelop the patient with care and concern. Within the confines of this traditional cluster of moral and social expectations, physicians and family members should seek to ensure appropriate medical care.

In sum, the family functions as a strong social support system in times of sickness. This support can be cultivated by the physician as a strong ally in the caring aspects of medicine. As the central social unit, the family is the anchor of Filipino society; it affects all aspects of life, as well as every decision an individual makes, including those about health care.

Note

1. A distinction is drawn between persons in authority who have the right to settle a controversy—as a judge can make a ruling—and those who are authorities in the sense of *experts*.

References

Andres, T. 1985. *Filipino Values*. Manila: Our Lady of Manaoag Publisher.

Kuan, L. H. 1976. Concept of health care and illness. Master's thesis presented at University of the Philippines.

Mendez, P. P., et al. 1984. *The Filipino Family in Transition*. Manila: Centro Escolar University, Research and Development Center.

The Family versus the Individual: Family Planning[1]

Angeles Tan Alora, Danilo Tiong, and
Josephine M. Lumitao

All societies throughout history have upheld the importance and value of the family. Although the family is as old as humanity itself, different cultures have different customs, traditions, taboos, beliefs, and superstitions about the family. They give importance to the family in different ways. Many religions also value the family, although the doctrinal and moral reasons for doing so differ. Nevertheless, the family is important and valuable in all traditional societies and religions.

Several factors may explain the universal valuation of the family. First, the family is the nucleus of society. Second, an individual's identity is very much connected with the family. Third, individuals have a sense of belonging to their families. Fourth, as is often the case in the developing world, families are the source of social and economic security for poor Filipinos. In the past, having more family members (i.e., more children) has meant greater resources for the family. In particular, this philosophy guaranteed support for the aged. For all these reasons, the family is the social unit of greatest importance and value for Filipinos. It provides Filipinos with emotional security, economic support, and a deep sense of belonging.

Today, all understandings of the family are set within worldwide debates regarding population control and limitations on the size of the family. Many international agencies confront developing nations in general, and the Philippines in particular, with the need to limit population growth. On close examination, different manifestations and expressions of this awareness reveal conflicting but related values. Secular and religious leaders are on all sides of the debate. Each group speaks its own language in the sense that it uses its own terminology such that others do not fully understand them. Each side has its own views, reasons, convictions, and beliefs that support its own conclusions.

The Roman Catholic Church, the largest religious body in the Philippines, has been consistent in its teaching on responsible parenthood and birth control. This position is based on the inseparable connection willed by God between the two meanings of the conjugal act: the unitive and procreative meanings. It also regards as intrinsically immoral every action that in anticipation of the conjugal act, in its accomplishment, or in the development of its natural consequences proposes—as an end or a means—to render procreation impossible. Thus, all artificial methods of limiting the number of children are considered immoral.

Social and economic conditions in the Philippines, however, make raising an unlimited number of children well nigh impossible. Given parents' moral obligation to feed, clothe, shelter, educate, and love the children they beget, the average Filipino couple finds itself in a very difficult situation.

This essay presents the conflicting values of this complex situation. It describes the tensions between the teachings of the Roman Catholic Church and the family planning programs of the Philippines. It also considers the following factors: the role of the culture, with its emphasis on the value of family and children; *pakikisama* resulting in the formation of *barkada;* the machismo image of the Filipino male, expressed in an abundant number of children; the social and economic situation; and the Western influence on women seeking to assert their individuality and find personal fulfillment.

The Role of Culture

Limiting the number of children is a goal that Filipinos find difficult to accept. In religion classes, they are taught that marriage is primarily for procreation. Children are gifts from God who bring good luck, happiness, and emotional security. Children bind couples and inspire them to work more and lead moral lives. They assure continuance of the family name. They are economic investments, especially for poor families. They form a social support system and insurance in old age. Many children means more family members to work on the farm, to earn money, and to care for their parents when the parents are elderly. Both sexes are valued: the male to be a breadwinner, the female to care for the home. Children are a public testimony to the moral and pious lives of their parents. Large families are considered blessed; sterility and childlessness are pitied. Moreover, machismo is still very strong in the Filipino male, and siring a great number of children is a symbol of this machismo.

On the other hand, economic constraints, Western influences, and the feminist movement have affected Filipino culture, especially in the family. Although husbands and wives still have traditional roles—the husband as breadwinner and the wife primarily as homemaker (although she may have full-time employment)—because of the present economic situation, and occasionally for personal fulfillment, most families need two sources of income to live comfortably. A working wife contributes to the family's income and may even help support her parents and siblings. She is not totally dependent on her husband. Regardless of the reasons for the Filipino wife's employment, this additional role affects the relationship with her husband and children. This dynamic has significant effects that are even more evident and significant when the wife works abroad.

The Filipino male is the symbolic head of the family; he establishes its unity and its identity. The primary role of the Filipino husband is that of provider. As symbolic head and leader of the family, the Filipino husband is expected to establish and develop relationships outside the family. The Filipino view of *pakikisama* encourages him to form associations outside the family in his *barkada* (peer group). When the husband spends more time with his *barkada* because of *pakikisama* (especially in the form of drinking sprees after office hours), marital problems may ensue. When both parents are working and pursuing their own interests, there is insufficient time for bonding and communication between spouses. This situation is not ideal for the practice of natural methods of family planning because opportune times and moments of affectional disposition may not coincide.

Reasons for Family Planning

Demographers insist on population control. They claim that the world's resources cannot cope with the alarming population increase: Unabated human population growth threatens the environment, as well as humans' ability to feed themselves adequately.

The Philippine population in 1995 was 68,614,162; the growth rate was 2.32 percent. The total labor force was 28,040,000, and there were 2,342,000 unemployed Filipinos. The Philippines and the Filipino people are poor. The 1995 gross domestic product (GDP) was 802,866 million pesos; in 1996, GDP increased to 848,451 million pesos. Per capita income in 1995 was 20,093 pesos (about US$772) (National Statistical Commission Board 1997).

There also are many individual and familial reasons to limit the number of children. For medical reasons, a woman may be advised not to get pregnant. An existing illness may be exacerbated, therapy for a life-threatening disease may contraindicate pregnancy, or a genetic disorder may result in an abnormal child. Personal reasons also may influence a woman's decision to delay having children or not to have a child, such as a previous traumatic pregnancy or delivery, a high-pressure period in her career or life, or working abroad to earn more money.

In 1989, 300 married adults, ages 16–47 years, were asked to list their reasons for limiting the number of children they had. Their responses (which were not limited to one choice) were as follows: economics, 199 (66.3 percent); difficult times, 119 (39.7 percent); health, 49 (16.3 percent); difficult births, 15 (5.0 percent); to give enough attention to existing children, 15 (5.0 percent); ideal family size, 9 (3.0 percent); financial dependence on parents, 6 (2.0 percent); already having a child, 5 (1.7 percent); and figure consciousness, 2 (0.7 percent). Overwhelmingly, the primary reason for limiting the number of children is the financial situation of the couple (Health Act Information Network 1991; South-East Asian Center for Bioethics 1990).

For environmental, financial, medical, or personal reasons, when there appear to be too many children or children too close in age for married couples to fulfill their responsibility of rearing the children properly, couples resort to various means of planned parenthood.

Choice of Family Planning Methods

In a study on family planning attitudes among Filipinos (Alora et al. 1991), the methods cited by 300 couples to prevent or limit pregnancy were as follows: natural family planning (rhythm), 90 (30.0 percent); pills, 80 (26.66 percent); tubal ligation, 39 (13.0 percent); withdrawal, 27 (9.0 percent); intrauterine device (IUD), 16 (5.33 percent); abstinence, 10 (3.33 percent); condom/diaphragm, 9 (3 percent); others or a combination of methods, 29 (9.7 percent). The reasons for choosing not to use natural family planning were ignorance, 50 (22.2 percent); ineffectiveness, 75 (33.3 percent); difficulty, 83 (36.88 percent); religion, 3 (1.33 percent); irregular menstrual period, 9 (4.0 percent); and irregular schedule of being together, 4 (1.77 percent).

These data show that only 30 percent of the couples use natural family planning methods, whereas 53.99 percent use artificial methods, and 13 percent resorted to tubal ligation. This dichotomy in the supposedly official morality (i.e., natural family planning) and the predominant practice of birth control could be attributed to several factors.

The Philippines Family Planning Program (1990–1994), in its fifth guideline, enumerates equally all of the means available to couples for family planning, including natural family planning, IUDs, oral contraceptives, and sterilization. Although the Catholic Bishops Conference of the Philippines reiterates its objection to contraceptives and sterilization and seeks a greater emphasis on natural family planning, the Church's effort and education campaign on natural family planning is minimal compared with the widespread and abundant resources available for artificial methods of birth control. Health centers all over the country are staffed by some rural health care physicians but predominantly by midwives who are given incentives (a point system that converts to financial rewards) when they are able to recruit people who will use an artificial method. Couples also receive incentives. Males who undergo vasectomy receive a transistor radio. Tubal ligations are performed without charge. Because economic constraints are a perennial problem for most couples, these inducements can be very strong. Statistics from the Family Planning Service of the Department of Health show that in 1995, new recruits for artificial birth control totaled 829,425, and continuous users totaled 3,239,657—for a total of 4,069,482 users of artificial methods of family planning. Some of these agencies regularly conduct provincial trips to far-flung towns to perform tubal ligations and vasectomies. Foreign funding and widespread advertisement on Filipino mass media (including television advertising about the use of condoms and the pill) contribute to greater information about and public knowledge of artificial methods.

Failure with natural family planning is common. Many couples remain ignorant about how to use it properly. The inherent difficulty in explaining the method involved in natural family planning and the mutual efforts required on the part of the couple to make it successful provide a further advantage to artificial methods that require minimal explanation (if any). Natural family planning requires periodic abstinence, which can be extremely difficult. For example, when one family member works far away and comes home only for a few weeks or months, abstinence during that time is extremely difficult. The husband may insist on having intercourse, whereas the wife, who may want to avoid another child, may refuse. As a result, she may be tempted to use artificial contraception to satisfy her husband's sexual needs and avoid the conception of another child. Many Filipinos believe that a wife's refusal to have sexual intercourse with her husband is a sufficient reason for the husband to take a mistress.

Another contributory factor is the fact that, of the 28 medical schools in the country, only 5 are Catholic schools where natural family planning is emphasized. Of the 122 hospitals approved for internship and residency training programs, only 4 are Catholic hospitals that teach natural family planning and forbid sterilization procedures. This disparity between the resources (financial, staffing, health care institutions) available for artificial methods and those for natural family planning is significant. The Roman Catholic Church became aware of this gap and in 1996 started parish-based programs to teach natural family planning. Nevertheless, the Church's resources are minimal compared to those available for persons who are proselytizing artificial methods.

One might think that in a predominantly Roman Catholic country such as the Philippines there would be an inherent focus on natural family planning; in fact, however, most resources are secular—and they emphasize artificial means of birth control. This paradox reveals a tension between the predominant Roman Catholic morality of the culture and the way birth control is actually conducted. This tension is manifest between patients and health care providers and between health care workers and health care institutions (Catholic Physician's Guild of the Philippines 1993).

For many Filipinos, religion means going to church and participating in various religious rites. It does not necessarily mean living faithfully according to Catholic moral teachings. A Filipino couple may practice withdrawal or use a condom or diaphragm. The wife may take contraceptives or undergo tubal ligation, yet continue to fulfill other religious duties. The family will go to Sunday mass and receive the sacraments with no qualms of conscience. Couples rationalize that the graver sin is having many children they cannot support—or resorting to abortion if natural family planning fails. They justify their use of artificial contraception as a choice of the lesser evil. There often is a significant cultural gulf between Filipinos who live their lives within the context of the Roman Catholic faith and those who have been secularized to various degrees.

Moreover, poor people in the Philippines have less motivation to limit the number of their children. This attitude is quite understandable from the perspective of the social support system, in which children serve as insurance for old age. When one is poor, having more children is a prudent strategy. This manner of reasoning should not be condemned but understood as a survival tactic. The result is that religious and economic concerns favor large families.

The Formation of Conscience

Saying "follow your conscience" in choosing a family planning method can be very misleading. Instead, the couple should follow an *informed conscience*. This informed conscience requires discernment and varies according to the gravity of the moral problem or choice presented. Couples are expected to consult, reflect, and examine issues, using the teachings of the Church in the situation in which they find themselves. Nevertheless, the issue of whether to disturb the good faith of a patient/couple using artificial contraception is another delicate area that calls for discernment. A Roman Catholic physician may find that a Catholic patient is ignorant of the Church's prohibition of tubal ligation and have grounds for not disturbing that ignorance.

Respect for the conscience of the health care worker is expected in all situations. These workers should not be pressured to perform or be engaged in actions they consider immoral. Authoritarian Catholic health care givers who are secularized will be a problem in this regard, however, for patients and for health care workers. In cases in which the law (e.g., legalized abortion) is in conflict with their moral convictions, a "conscience clause" should offer realistic protection to health care workers without prejudicing their career or professional reputation. In fact, however, circumstances may be much more difficult.

Much happens that ought not occur according to the official dominant morality and bioethics. Some Filipino cultural characteristics might conflict with obligations in conscience; for example, a couple may agree to tubal ligation out of respect for the health worker (an authority figure), whom they will not contradict because of submissiveness or *hiya*. A teenage girl may accept her mother's decision to have an abortion because of submissiveness and *hiya*, as well as to prevent scandal to the family.

Because the population problem is a socioeconomic issue, the Church and the state have obligations to address them. Still, neither can decide for the couple or impose a decision. They can only issue guidelines. The individual couple has the responsibility to make its own decision regarding the number of children to have, when to have them, and what method of birth regulation to use. They have the obligation to seek correct information, to consider different options, and to choose the option that is in accord with their conscience. Most often, however, the larger amount of resources focused on artificial methods of birth control affects the decision of couples, leading to a dissonance with the morality most officially hold.

Illustrative Cases

CASE 1: Anna, a 23-year-old nurse who is single and a graduate of a Catholic university, is the eldest of four children. She applied and was accepted as an operating room nurse in the department of obstetrics and gynecology of a tertiary care government hospital. Anna felt very lucky to have been accepted because of the prestige of the hospital and because of the higher pay. She needed the extra money to support her brother, who was in his second year of college. She knew that tubal ligations and IUD insertions were done very often in the hospital, but fortunately she was able to ask her supervisor that she not be asked to assist in these procedures. Anna had learned in school that these procedures are not morally allowed. One day, however, Dr. Bacay (a Catholic who was the head of the department and a graduate of the state university) scheduled a tubal ligation. Because of the number of patients, Anna was scheduled to assist. She asked for permission not to assist because of religious beliefs, but Dr. Bacay got angry, accused her of insubordination, and threatened to report her to the head of the nursing service—his close friend—if Anna refused.

ANALYSIS: This case illustrates the difficulties encountered by Catholic health care workers who work in government hospitals. Although the Philippines is predominantly Catholic, varying degrees of secularization among health care workers and health care institutions give rise to moral tensions and conflicts. Anna is placed in a very difficult situation because of her need for the extra salary, compounded by the threat of being reported to her superior (with the possibility of expulsion). The fact that Anna spoke her mind and refused to assist Dr. Bacay, the department head and a formidable authority figure, is remarkable. Most health care workers who faced such a problem would simply keep quiet and do one of two things: resign from the hospital, or stop resisting and assist in procedures with varying degrees of guilt, expressing criticism periodically in forums of Catholic health care workers. Most nurses would have recourse to the latter action because of a combination of several factors: cultural emphasis on the authority figure of physicians, financial need, and pervasive and increasing secularization in the medical field.

CASE 2: Mr. and Mrs. Consing, both of whom are in their early thirties and are practicing Catholics, have five children. All of their babies were delivered by Dr. Bondoc. Mrs. Consing is an office worker; her husband is a high school teacher. Their combined salary is P8,000 ($325) per month. They pay a monthly rent of P3,500 ($135). Both feel that five children is enough for them. They heard in church that natural family planning is the only method of birth control that is morally allowed. They have occasional difficulty with natural family planning, but so far they have managed well. Dr. Bondoc advises Mrs. Consing to have a tubal ligation because they have already completed their family. Moreover, the procedure is very practical: It is a one-time procedure that lasts about 15–20 minutes. Furthermore, if they have no money, Dr. Bondoc could refer them to a center where the procedure is performed *gratis*. Mr. and Mrs. Consing are confused because they know that Dr. Bondoc is a Roman Catholic.

ANALYSIS: This case illustrates the pressures on an average-income couple exerted by the financial burden of rearing a moderately large family, especially when a method of family planning is made available to them, contrary to their moral commitments, by a health care giver whom they thought to be a moral friend but who has proved to be a moral stranger. The incentives for Mr. and Mrs. Consing to choose tubal ligation are considerable. There is no cost, and it is practical and easy. In addition, it bears the endorsement of an authority figure, Dr. Bondoc, who delivered their five children. All of these factors may be too much for the couple to resist. Most couples would simply agree with the authoritarian health care giver who advocates an efficient and practical method, without further thought about its moral implications. This increasing secularization is a very powerful force with which practicing Roman Catholics must learn to contend. Moreover, it engenders a battle in a culture war between the traditional Filipino morality and the emerging secular morality in the Philippines.

CASE 3: Mrs. Dizon is a 30-year-old laundry woman who has been pregnant four times and has three live children, who now range in age from one to six years old. Mrs. Dizon's husband earns tips parking cars. Mr. and Mrs. Dizon do not want any more children. Their combined irregular income ranges from P1,000 to P1,500 monthly ($40–60). They live in a rented room and have barely enough food, water, and clothing. Both try to live faithfully according to Roman Catholic teachings. They have refused a vasectomy and a tubal ligation. They ask Dr. Egay for help in limiting the number of their children. After Mrs. Dizon's fourth cesarean section for the birth of yet another child, Dr. Egay finds the uterus to be "thin." She chooses to do a hysterectomy. Is her action ethical?

ANALYSIS: This question is a serious one for any Catholic physician who chooses to live in accordance with Catholic teachings. It presents the physician with a cluster of considerations that are unknown to many religions.

In this case, the focus is on the diagnostic finding: "On cesarean section, the uterus is found to be thin." If a competent obstetrician assesses the extent of uterine "thinness" to be a medical risk, the uterus should be removed, based on the principle of totality: If an organ is diseased, it may be removed to preserve the total health, as well as the life, of a person. This decision is justified on the basis that a pathologic uterus is being removed for the good of the patient, with regard for the circumstances of a large family, the patient's request for help, and the individual values of the physician. This chain of reasoning captures the actual clinical context of a great deal of gynecological medicine in the Philippines, given a devout Roman Catholic frame of reference.

Often, however, assessment of uterine thinness is not entirely objective. Given the same case, different obstetricians may arrive at different conclusions, based on their own personal values: concern for overpopulation, commitment to strict Catholic teachings, eagerness to respond to a patient's request, compassion for the couple. This case illustrates the truth that many decisions happen in "gray areas" where boundaries can easily shift or change. Physicians often find themselves in gray areas where different factors can legitimately be given different rankings. Even the understanding of risk is relative. In such cases, the physician easily may find himself or herself deciding in favor of the factor the physician considers to be more important for nonmedical reasons. The competing claims of religious beliefs, financial needs, and secular mores will continue to exert their influence on decisions in shaping the ways decisions are made in Filipino gynecological medicine. The character of the decision will not be understandable outside the special, compelling moral forces that are vying to direct the construction of this area of medical reality.

Conclusion

In the Philippines, population control is a complex problem that can be understood only in terms of the competitive interplay of several competing moral visions. Filipino culture, with its emphasis on the family as a social support system, resists family planning, yet financial constraints and an emerging secular mores dictate otherwise. A tension arises within the culture between the official traditional morality and the predominant secular morality, with its accepted practice of birth control. The increasing secularization of available resources will cause the fault lines between traditional and post-traditional Filipino culture to become increasingly unstable. This instability, and the conflicts it will engender, will be manifested in the lives of health care workers, in interactions between patients and health care workers, and in communication between health care workers and institutions. Health care practitioners will find their moral integrity challenged and their moral vision brought into question.

Note

1. This essay uses *natural family planning* and *the rhythm method* as equivalent terms, although in theory they are different methods to avoid unwanted preganancy. For many authors, the rhythm method identifies only a general attention to dates after the previous menstrual cycle when a woman is least likely to be fertile. The equivocation in this essay illustrates the general conflation of these methods in developing nations.

References

Alora, A. et al. (eds.). 1991. *Casebook in Bioethics*. Manila: South-East Asian Center for Bioethics.

Catholic Physician's Guild of the Philippines. 1993. *Newsletter* (November).

Health Act Information Network. 1991. *Health Alert 7* (April-May).

National Statistical Commission Board. 1997. *Philippine Statistical Yearbook*. Makati City, The Philippines: National Statistical Commission Board.

South-East Asian Center for Bioethics. 1990, *Bioethics Newsletter* (November).

Care of the Elderly

Victoria Pusung

In traditional societies, the family takes for granted values such as obligation, honor, and caring. Traditions in the Filipino culture underscore the importance of *utang na loob*: that children and grandchildren will never allow their aging parents and close relatives to be neglected.

Elderly Filipinos live with the family. They are cared for until they die, and family support includes the provision of health care. This tradition is ingrained in each child; all Filipino children grow with this concept in their hearts. This attitude is regarded as a sort of moral reciprocity: When the children were young, the parents gave their energies and their time to raise and educate them; now, when they are adults, it is their turn to take care of their parents. In this way, the concept of *utang na loob* is perpetuated, and the failings of *walanghiya* are avoided. This caring tradition lives on among Filipino families, and younger generations are expected to carry it on in perpetuity.

The Role of the Elderly in the Filipino Family

The role of the elderly as patriarchs and matriarchs of the family encompasses many other roles. Perhaps because of the high degree of filial honor and respect accorded to the elderly, old age passes uneventfully. There are no reports that elderly parents and grandparents are passing their latter years in crisis, depression, or loneliness. In a survey conducted by Letty G. Kuan in 1984–1985 among retired members of the government service and the social security system, the 100 respondents, ranging in age from 76 to 83, defined their role in the family as follows:

- They cement family bonds. Through family reunions, children and grandchildren endeavor to come together, and the elderly unify the family ties.
- Their presence makes the younger generation reflect on their actions and reactions. Because elders call attention to improper behavior by younger family members, elders see their role as guides for good manners and right conduct.

- They play the role of seasoned and wise advisers who view things with more maturity and wisdom. Hence, they become family counselors.
- They transmit ancestral values and the history of the origin of the family name. The presence of the elderly induces younger family members to trace the origin of the family name—widening the family circle by identifying other relatives.
- They act as the caretakers, property watchers, and babysitters for the grandchildren. Married adult children are relieved of stress by having aging parents at home because the parents take care of the house while the adult children are at work. Grandparents are devoted babysitters for the grandchildren. Grandparents demonstrate affection, which is reciprocated by the grandchildren. Grandchildren listen to their grandparents because the parents are at work and do not have as much time for interaction with the grandchildren as the grandparents do.

Illustrative Cases

CASE 1: Lolo is an 84-year-old married male who suffered a myocardial infarction. He was discharged in improved condition, but he required long-term rehabilitation. Lolo's children shouldered responsibility for his hospital and medical bills. On discharge, a son took the responsibility of bringing Lolo to the rehabilitation clinic in the morning; a grandson volunteered to bring him home. One married daughter moved into Lolo's house, along with her husband and three children, so she could personally take care of both parents. All of Lolo's married children continued to share the financial needs of their parents. Every Saturday and Sunday, five of his married children entertained him with their stories about school and their accomplishments. Lolo always looked forward to these visits, and even after he recovered, these visits continued.

ANALYSIS: For Filipinos, the family is the primary social support, as well as an insurance system in times of need, aging, and illness. The family feels concern, which is more marked when an aging parent is ill.

CASE 2: An 83-year-old single female suffering from chronic obstructive lung disease refuses to continue taking food and medications because she feels that she is a burden to her niece. She lives with her niece, who regards caring for her aunt as her duty—not only because her aunt sent her to college but also because the aunt took care of her from birth.

ANALYSIS: With advancing age, a role reversal often takes place. In families in which the aged becomes dependent on adult relations, this dependence can bring about lowered morale, as well as pleas for reassurance. Hence, the niece recognizes and accepts her *utang na loob* from her aunt, to whom she gives physical as well as emotional support.

CASE 3: Mrs. S. is a 72-year-old widow with chronic leukemia. During the past four years, she has been repeatedly admitted to the hospital for chemo-therapy and blood transfusions. A few days ago, she developed fever and diarrhea and rapidly grew weak. She was readmitted to the hospital, but her condition deteriorated in spite of the treatment. Mrs. S.'s physician feels that her immunosuppressed condition makes her susceptible and that the infection is permanent. In addition, a remission of her leukemia is not a reasonable ex-pectation. Mrs. S. is terminally ill. Mrs. S. has been aware of the severity of her illness for the past two years. She expresses her wish that no additional treat-ment be given; she says that she is prepared to die. Her oldest daughter, who is working overseas, calls the physician and begs that her mother be kept alive until her return within the week.

ANALYSIS: In this case, the elderly parent does not wish to be a burden to her family. At the same time, she faces and accepts the reality of her condi-tion. The daughter's request can be interpreted as a desire to bid good-bye to a beloved parent, given the importance of obligations of children to their par-ents. This use of resources becomes appropriate. Moreover, the mother finds herself vested with an obligation to stay alive to make possible a last meeting.

CASE 4: Dr. Lopez was consulted by Mr. Reyes because of jaundice and a right upper quadrant mass. After a series of examinations, Dr. Lopez made a diagnosis of hepatic carcinoma. Mr. Reyes's family asked Dr. Lopez not to tell Mr. Reyes of his disease. Dr. Lopez, however—having been trained in the West and convinced of the benefits of truth-telling and patient autonomy—never-theless told Mr. Reyes of his condition. Upon learning of this development, Mr. Reyes's family was very upset and took Dr. Lopez off the case.

ANALYSIS: Several Filipino cultural characteristics were violated:

- Authority: The family takes over decision making for the sick person. They decide what he should or should not be told; their authority was violated.
- Bad news is never given directly. Dr. Lopez told Mr. Reyes of his ter-minal cancer.
- *Pakikisama.* The family asked Dr. Lopez not to tell Mr. Reyes of his condition and expected him to follow their wishes. Dr. Lopez did not accede to their request.

To the Western bioethicist, the case of Mr. Reyes and Dr. Lopez may seem unbelievable. Even Dr. Lopez was surprised at the family's action. Cultural prohibitions were not taught in medical school. He made a serious cultural mistake that was unrelated to scientific health care: He violated the norms of traditional Filipino bioethics. In caring for the sick, and even more so the elderly sick, the family assumes all decision-making authority. Dr. Lopez may be a very competent physician, but unless he also is sensitive to cultural norms and the requirements of Filipino bioethics, he will not be a popular one.

PART III

The Health Care Team

Professional Relationships in Health Care

Antonio Cabezon, O.P., Edna G. Monzon, and
Angelica Francisco

Health care delivery is a team effort. It requires harmonious relationships within the team and is directed toward the patient's best interest. Therefore, the team should maintain a collegial relationship; team members should respect one another's complementary and diverse expertise, listen to one another, and show solidarity. Without these relationships, their common mission will suffer.

Administrators and attending physicians are recognized as authorities to be respected and obeyed. In the health care team, the consultant holds the highest rank, followed by the fellows, residents, interns, clerks, and medical students. Within the team, the attending physician is the leader, and nurses and other allied health care givers are subordinates.

The lower-ranking members of the team obey because they consider the consultant to be authoritative when he or she demonstrates appropriate knowledge and expertise. A problem arises when the consultant is perceived to be merely authoritarian; as such, the consultant is obeyed only because of his or her official position, combined with the fear of sanctions imposed by the consultant for criticism, noncompliance, or disobedience. Occasionally, subordinates may feel that they have a legitimate disagreement, suggestion, or point of view that should be considered, yet they keep silent because of fear and *hiya*.

Because Filipinos generally are nonconfrontational, they tend toward nonadversarial approaches. Out of *hiya* (respect for authority) or *pakikisama*, they choose not to question authority. On the other hand, the person in authority may abuse and misuse his or her power and position.[1]

Competition within the medical community may be helpful if health care providers are challenged to do their best, but success may give rise to envy, jealousy, and other problems. One may try to outdo another at the other's expense or do something to put the other person down (what Filipinos call "crab mentality").

The common features of Filipino social behavior that play an important role in inter- and intraprofessional relationships are *hiya*, *pakikisama*, submissiveness or respect for authority, *kababang loob* (humility), *utang na loob*, and crab mentality.

CASE 1: Mr. Santos is admitted to the hospital because of abdominal full-ness and progressive loss of weight. He is diagnosed with liver cancer. The con-sultant performs a blind liver biopsy; a few hours afterwards, the patient goes into shock and dies. The family asks the resident what the cause of death was. The consultant instructs the resident not to give any information.

ANALYSIS: Physicians commonly offer several reasons for not disclosing serious mistakes to patients or family. Most often, because many individuals are involved in patient care, responsibility is somewhat blurred; thus, it will be dif-ficult for one caregiver to acknowledge that he or she was at fault. Patients will lose their trust and may even sue the health care provider(s) in court. Moreover, colleagues and supervisors who are told of the mistake may be punitive rather than supportive. Nevertheless, determining the cause of mistakes is necessary for good quality care, as well as to prevent repetition of such mistakes.

In this particular case, the consultant is the authority, and he is in authority. Although the resident knows the cause of death, he or she will remain silent out of respect and fear of punishment that may affect his or her future.

CASE 2: Manay, a Roman Catholic medical intern, is assigned to a govern-ment hospital. She is assigned to assist in a cesarean section. When the section is over, she notes that the obstetrician is doing a tubal ligation, which is not in-cluded in the schedule, nor in the consent signed by the patient. Manay asks for permission to scrub out but is not allowed to do so.

ANALYSIS: Manay wants to leave because she is opposed to the tubal liga-tion. This situation is common for Roman Catholic trainees who are assigned to secular hospitals. Although there is an agreement to respect religious con-viction (a "conscience clause"), some consultants disregard it and instead im-pose sanctions that eventually affect the trainees' professional development. Trainees obey out of fear and respect for authority. Some, however, may fol-low their conscience and leave—and suffer the consequences of their action (see Appelbaum and Roth 1983; Faden 1989; Mazur 1986). Remarkably, from the perspective of Western bioethics, moral attention is focused on the fact that the operation performed was unnatural from a religious point of view (i.e., sur-gical sterilization), not the fact that the operation was performed without the consent of the patient.

CASE 3: Miss Sandoval, a nurse in the emergency room, is very busy at-tending to victims of a vehicular accident, most of whom require blood trans-fusions. One of the patients who is transfused develops severe reactions because he is given the wrong blood type. Miss Sandoval tells the attending physician of her mistake. She is told to keep quiet and remove the blood immediately. With feelings of remorse, she telephones her supervisor for help but is reprimanded instead. Because of feelings of guilt, she tells the relatives of her mistake. When the administrator learns about this confession, Miss Sandoval is suspended.

ANALYSIS: Mistakes do happen. When they do, who is going to shoulder the responsibility? The nurse admits that the blood mixup was her fault, but should this error be disclosed, and if so, who should do it? Did Miss Sandoval act rightly in disclosing her mistake to the family?

Disclosure of mistakes, especially when they are serious, imposes tremendous problems for the physician and the hospital. In this particular case, will the attending physician assume responsibility as team leader? Most physicians would offer reasons for not disclosing mistakes to patients or family: They will lose trust, they may get angry, and they may even sue in court. Moreover, colleagues and supervisors who are told of such mistakes may be punitive rather than supportive, as in this case. On the other hand, nondisclosure may not help the person learn, much less prevent recurrences of such mistakes.

What should have been done? The attending physician, the nurse involved, and the supervisor should have discussed it first, and the nurse's emotional remorse should have been acknowledged.

CASE 4: Mrs. Itchon, a 42-year-old multigravida, is admitted to the hospital because of spotting. She is advised to undergo diagnostic curettage to rule out cancer, to which she consents. The histopathological report shows chorionic villi—which is suggestive of pregnancy. Dr. Fajardo, the obstetrician-gynecologist, calls Dr. Lopez, the pathologist, to change the official report. Dr. Fajardo is the consultant who sends Dr. Lopez the most referrals.

ANALYSIS: Dr. Lopez is in a quandary about whether to accede to his friend's request out of *pakikisama* or *utang na loob* or to follow his religious convictions, remain honest, and preserve his integrity (see Stark 1989; Todd and Horan 1989). The case illustrates the disinclination to report negligence (i.e., the failure to perform a pregnancy test prior to the procedure), as well as the felt obligation to falsify reports to meet personal obligations.

CASE 5: Dr. Suapang, a well-known, 50-year-old practitioner, enjoys attending international medical conferences. He uses these conferences as opportunities to learn, as well as to obtain needed rest and recreation. His attendance is sponsored by a pharmaceutical company.

ANALYSIS: The physician and the drug industry serve patients' best interest, albeit in different ways. The physician prescribes the best drug for his or her patient, and the industry provides this drug. Unlike other enterprises, in which the consumer chooses which product to buy, in the health care delivery system physicians choose the product. They prescribe the drug, and the consumer/patient purchases it. The physician determines the movement of a product in the pharmaceutical market. The industry needs the physician to prescribe, so medical practitioners are the focus of drug companies' promotional activities.

In the Philippines, pharmaceutical agents often support continuing medical education activities. They also treat physicians to meals; subsidize physician attendance at local and international meetings; distribute gifts such as pens, notepads, and even clinic furniture and equipment; and provide entertainment and other forms of hospitality.

Pharmaceutical companies' support for continuing medical education is commendable. Improvement of physicians' knowledge leads to better health care. Yet we cannot ignore the fact that these "giveaways" are paid for by patients. To what extent do the costs of promotional activities add to the cost of drugs? This issue is especially significant in developing countries where most of the population is poor and unable to buy medicine. The Filipino physician can be the most caring at the bedside, yet the medical community has shown apathy to social issues that involve patient welfare. Moreover, inasmuch as the patients pay for the physicians' education, should the patients be informed?

Another concern is the extent to which receiving these "giveaways" affects a physician's prescribing habits. *Pakikisama* and *utang na loob* are cultural givens that demand return for favors. The patients' best interest is not served when a physician prescribes less than the best to repay a favor previously received (see American College of Physicians 1998; Brisker 1987; Connelly and Fallermurn 1988; Morreim 1989; Relman 1989; Royal College of Physicians 1986).

A third concern is the extent to which these activities actually improve physicians' knowledge. Many presentations are purely promotional and are biased toward a particular product. At conventions and international conferences, many physicians spend time touring, socializing, and shopping rather than attending scientific sessions.

Each physician must take on the responsibility of reviewing his or her relationship with the industry. This assessment is part of the physician's continuing responsibility to his or her patients. Each pharmaceutical company must take on the responsibility of reviewing its offers to physicians. This review is part of its continuing responsibility to justice.

Note

1. There is a distinction between someone who *is* an authority—an expert in a particular field—and someone who is *in* authority and thus has the right to settle a controversy (e.g., a judge).

References

American College of Physicians. 1998. Ethics manual. *Annals of Internal Medicine* 128: 576–94.

Appelbaum, P. S., and L. H. Roth. 1983. Patients who refuse treatment in the medical hospital. *Journal of the American Medical Association* 250, 1296–1301.

Brisker, E. M. 1987. Industrial marketing and medical ethics. *New England Journal of Medicine* 320: 1690–92.

Connelly, J. E., and S. Fallermurn. 1988. Ethical problems in the medical office. *Journal of the American Medical Association* 260: 812–15.

Faden, R. 1989. Enforcing informed consent requirements: Form or substance. *Journal of the American Medical Association* 261: 1948–49.

Mazur, D. J. 1986. What patients must be told prior to a medical procedure. *American Journal of Medicine* 81: 1051–54.

Morreim, E. H. 1989. Conflict of interest: Profits and problems in physician referrals. *Journal of the American Medical Association* 262: 390–94.

Relman, A. S. 1989. Economic incentives in clinical investigation. *New England Journal of Medicine* 320: 933–34.

Royal College of Physicians. 1986. The relationship between physicians and the pharmaceutical industry. *Journal of the Royal College of Physicians* 20: 235–42.

Stark, F. H. 1989. Physicians' conflicts in patient referrals. *Journal of the American Medical Association* 262: 397–98.

Todd, J. S., and J. K. Horan. 1989. Physician referrals: The AMA Review. *Journal of the American Medical Association* 262: 385–86.

Conscience and Health Care Practices: The Case of the Philippines

Letty G. Kuan and Tamerlane Lana, O.P.

A young Catholic priest from Manila, about to relax after an exhausting day, receives a call from a confused mother inquiring about the morality of contraception. The mother says that she knows her Catholic doctrine, yet she cannot reconcile it with her marital and family conditions. Her family, she claims, is hard up economically and cannot afford another mouth to feed. She and her husband have tried to employ natural means of birth control, but their methods have been ineffective, so they also have tried artificial means. Yet she expresses the desire to remain faithful to Catholic teaching. Obviously tired and half-asleep, the priest asks point-blank whether she really knows her doctrine, to which the woman answers in the affirmative. He hastily remarks, "Fine, then follow your conscience." She thanks him and then hangs up the phone.

The decision the woman takes as a result of the conversation must be a source of worry for the priest because he has given her hasty, ambiguous advice. We do not want to make a value judgment concerning his rash reply, however. We want to show in this case a typical example of how Filipinos value the role of conscience in their lives and how they desire to attain an informed conscience that can become the standard for their moral decisions. We also see in this case, however, a vivid example of a Filipino grappling with a conflict of conscience as she tries to compare her own personal judgment with the moral teaching of the Church. We deal with the typical Filipino conscience and its implications for health care practices. The following example may demonstrate how this conscience functions within the Filipino cultural setting.

A respectable columnist of a local newspaper recently made an interesting observation regarding the 46-member Committee of Congress, which deliberated on a move to impeach a government official whose position—which demands unsullied and unquestionable integrity and wisdom—was threatened by his involvement in an alleged bribery for political favor. There was an attempt, the writer said, to make an appeal to the committee members' *konsensyang Filipino*. Before the vote was cast, they endeavored to point out where the path of conscience lay, and they did so quite convincingly. Casting doubt on the integrity of the committee itself, the columnist remarked that to appeal to the congressmen's conscience is to assume that a congressman has one. Thankfully, he continued, that conscience is found in the nine committee members who opted not to follow the way of the 32 who flocked to the official's side. This observation is striking for its attempt to articulate a typically Filipino conscience, *konsensyang Filipino*. Is this conscience distinguishable from others of different cultures?

The newspaper columnist seems to imply that the Filipino lawmakers generally did not follow the path of that conscience. Yet these same people also may claim that they do follow the right path and even defend the rectitude of their own action. The congressmen may be convinced that the official was innocent, yet their action could be suspect because of a notable cultural factor: The decision might have been made because of *utang na loob* (gratitude) or *pakikisama* (loyalty to the person belonging to the group or party), which are very strong among Filipinos. Even if these cultural traits were determining factors in the lawmakers' decision, they would have to contend with the demands of justice dictated by their religion (predominantly Roman Catholic), which may lead to a conflict of conscience notwithstanding the claim that they have done the right thing. The columnist undoubtedly was judging the motivation and choice of the majority of congressmen according to his Catholic standards of justice and fairness. In this example, then, we could infer that the conscience of the Filipino appears simultaneously in the light of two powerful influences: the Catholic religion and authentically Filipino sociocultural norms. Not surprisingly, the Filipino often may find his or her conscience in conflict between these two factors. First, however, how is conscience generally understood?

The General Concept of Conscience

Conscience usually is associated with the "inner voice" that tells us what to do and not do and subsequently judges our actions. Some people may scoff at the notion that conscience is a personal inner voice, yet that voice speaks nonetheless. Doing things without "qualms of conscience" does not speak well of the person concerned. Yet such behavior is not as bad as not having a conscience at all. The ordinary Filipino recognizes this truth. A person without a conscience (in the native tongue, *walang budhi*) is a morally insensitive person who is not even bothered by immoral and inhuman actions.

Much of the Catholic tradition contributes to the Filipino understanding of conscience. Catholicism brings with it rich biblical themes that allude to the idea of conscience. St. Paul, for instance, calls conscience "the spiritual function," which is a personal and spontaneous reaction (2 Cor 5:11). It is a universal endowment of man (Rom 2:14), a "witness" by which one can point to the substance of the Law engraved in one's heart and with which one accuses and defends oneself—one's own inner mental dialogue (Rom 2:14-15). We can infer from this passage that although conscience can be considered radically personal, it is not a matter of an individual person's decisions. Conscience is a response to God's law, though it involves an individualized response. This Pauline notion of conscience and the law inspired the articulation of the responsibility of conscience in the Second Vatican Council's *Gaudium et spes (GS)*:

> Deep within his conscience man discovers a law which he has not laid upon himself but which he must obey. Its voice, ever calling him to love and to do what is good and to avoid evil, tells him inwardly at the right moment: do this, shun that. For man has in his heart a law inscribed by God. His dignity lies in observing this law, and by it he will be judged (GS 16).

In *Veritatis Splendor*, Pope John Paul II also reaffirmed the biblical fact that all persons are endowed with conscience and that conscience is witness to the individual's hidden desires, thoughts, plans, decisions, and actions. There, in the forum of conscience, each person should stand naked before God, affirming or condemning his or her own desires, thoughts, and acts. Earlier theologians who also were deeply spiritual regarded the innermost ground of conscience as the "spark of the soul." This "mysterious spiritual endowment" has been the object of philosophical study, especially in the field of Christian ethics. The nature and role of conscience have been thoroughly treated in this field.

In ethical reflections, conscience is considered in the broad sense as a moral faculty that makes known to each person his or her moral obligations and urges him or her to fulfill them. These promptings are definitely toward what are good, appropriate, and right courses of actions. Thus, when we refer to the path of conscience, we can only mean the right path. Because conscience shows what that path is, we usually regard it as cognitive: It is a faculty of knowing. That is why some people also call the conscience an awareness or recognition of what is right and wrong.

Yet the perception of what is right and wrong concretely takes place in particular situations that demand action. In those particular cases, the individual judges the rightness and wrongness of a course of action before and after it is performed; this judging obliges the individual to engage in or refrain from particular actions. Conformity or nonconformity to such judgments of conscience evokes either a sense of guilt or a sense of having acted properly. Concretely, in the Catholic tradition, conscience refers to the judgment of practical reason regarding the morality of a concrete action, obliging one to do the good and avoid what is evil. This understanding of conscience, however, is incomplete without looking at its link with the will and the feelings—the subject of moral virtues. Through their mediation, the moral faculty can function effectively. In other words, considering conscience merely as a perceptive faculty is inadequate. Many persons can distinguish right from wrong, yet this ability does not necessarily mean that they would follow their conscience and do what is right.

Following Bonaventure, conscience also can be understood as a volitive faculty, in the sense that the movement and empowerment of the will—and, under its command, the feelings—enable the individual to follow his or her best information and moral insights. This notion is in line with the Thomistic idea that "goodwill" must always accompany the judgment of conscience to enable us to do what is ethically good. This Catholic notion of conscience was shaped within Western thought and categories. Filipinos educated in Catholic morality often have translated it into their language and culture. In any event, Filipino Catholic students generally are exposed to this understanding of conscience.

The Filipino Concept of Conscience

In a local television commercial for a bath soap, a housewife is depicted as talking to her conscience. That conscience is her own self. This dialogue is portrayed vividly: The housewife is arguing with her reflection in the mirror. The self in the mirror is appealing to her to use the right kind of soap. The wife follows the advice. In the last scene of the commercial, the housewife is again speaking to herself in the mirror, this time thanking her self for the right advice. The presentation may appear to be superficial, yet even uneducated Filipinos easily recognize that other self as the housewife's *budhi*. This understanding of conscience reflects a peculiar orientation to reality, including oneself. Conscience is the other self—a deep thought that may not have an appeal to the Western analytic mind.

Interestingly, Filipinos would perceive that *budhi* in another way. It is found in the innermost core of mankind's being: *kalooban*. *Kalooban* may be roughly translated as the will. It is the seat of the individual's innermost thoughts and feelings as *hiya* (the peculiarly Filipino shame), *awa* (compassion), *malasakit* (care), *kabutihan* (goodness), *utang na loob* (gratitude), *budhi* (the locus of moral decisions)—inner traits that have significant bearings on health care decisions and practices. Thus, for Filipinos, conscience is related to the "heart," where one can relate with God and one's inner self rather than to the mind.

This discussion brings us to the fact that the Filipino perception of conscience is related to St. Paul's understanding of that universal endowment: a spiritual function that is deeply personal and serves as a witness of oneself. Filipinos are deeply religious people; thus, the *other self* that serves as their counselor, judge, and accuser is perceived to be standing always before the guidance and judgment of the unseen, personal God. When other people's lives are at stake, Filipinos feel responsible before God for the moral decisions they may make.

This belief explains Filipinos' peculiar moral sensitivity, which easily can be mistaken for vacillation in the process of decision and anxiety in "matter of life" decisions in health care settings. When a life-support system has to be withdrawn, health care providers will not easily or readily assume responsibility for doing the task. A physician may still feel responsible before God for the death of the patient after arriving at the decision to stop all support measures, even if he or she has diligently gone through the right procedures. "Maybe I should have done more to save the life of the patient" is not an unusual afterthought for a Filipino physician.

There are other ambiguities in the Filipino expression of conscience. Although a Filipino manifests moral sensitivity, his or her actions often contravene those moral convictions with a sense of resignation. This phenomenon makes sense only if we understand that, although the Catholic religion plays a significant role, the formation of Filipino conscience is culturally bound. The Introduction of this book discusses how these sociocultural norms contribute to the shaping of the Filipino conscience, often generating ambivalence in decisions and actions. One of the sources of Filipino culture is poverty, which drives people to opt for something that may contradict their moral and religious beliefs. A Filipino saying, *Kapit sa patalim* (roughly translated as "grabbing the knife by the blade"), vividly depicts this sad plight. If the young mother who is facing a dilemma regarding the issue of contraception indeed uses artificial means, her decision does not necessarily indicate a triumph of her individual conscience over the doctrine of the Church but an exigent, almost desperate response to poverty and deep concern for her family. We will not be surprised to find even devout and practicing Catholics who are tolerant of, if not sympathetic with, the mother's decision.

Family and religion are primary factors in the formation of the Filipino conscience from an early age. In this process, there is a clear emphasis on the role of lived experience and on exemplars of what a Filipino considers to be right and wrong, good and bad. These exemplars are provided by authority figures in the family (the parents), in the church (the priests), and in the school (academic mentors). We might say that the conscience of a Filipino is authoritarian—not necessarily in the sense of the Western standard as immature or ill-internalized but in the sense that a high regard for authority is a significant factor in the consideration of what is appropriate or inappropriate. In matters of morals, physicians readily consult the clergy, whom they consider to be authorities in the field. In bioethics rounds, health care professionals give more credence to priests than to the physicians themselves in the discussion of ethical issues.

In the health care setting, patients depend heavily on the judgment of the physicians because of their authoritative status in the society. Physicians, on the other hand, tend to demand submissiveness from patients, which more appropriately can be termed trust—not necessarily out of authoritarian arrogance but out of strong authoritative or paternalistic concerns for the patients. Physicians may not feel comfortable when patients incessantly pose questions regarding their condition. They would be regarded as *makulit*, an unflattering term for people who become overly persistent.

Family values and community ties that generate *pakikisama* (harmony with others) and *utang na loob* (gratitude) also play a significant role in Filipinos' moral judgments. Many cases in the medical setting offer evidence of the extent to which these family values influence decision making by patients and physicians. The case involving the deliberation of the ethical committee in Congress about an allegedly erring official is a function of the cultural values of *utang na loob* or *pakikisama* (sense of belonging to the same party). These norms may have become major factors bearing on the decision of the majority of the congressmen to side with the official accused of moral impropriety. The lawmakers might not easily admit that they have trodden the wrong path of conscience. In a parallel setting, physicians and patients may not easily admit that they have chosen the wrong course of action, given the many factors—mostly culturally bound—that influence their decision making.

Filipinos, then, are well aware of the role that conscience plays in their lives. Filipino health care providers are brought up in an atmosphere in which the family and Catholicism interplay, so generally they are, if not conscientious, at least conscious of the service dimension of the healing profession. Like many areas of the Filipino way of life, however, this orientation is being threatened by the profit-oriented culture that is rapidly invading Filipino society—a cause of concern for the medical and nursing schools in the country today.

This conscientiousness is the reason that many physicians and health care providers are anxious about being made collaborators in the performance of evil acts. The Catholic norm of legitimate cooperation in morally reprehensible acts undoubtedly still has great appeal for them because they know that this concept will relieve them of the burden of moral dilemmas in which they may find themselves. Traditional Catholic moral doctrine makes a distinction between formal and material cooperation through intention in the performance of an act. When the cooperator shares in the intention of the agent, the sin itself is willed and cooperation is formal. Otherwise, the cooperation is simply material. Material cooperation involves participation in the sinful act of another without sharing the intention to sin.

There are three different categories of material cooperation: immediate, mediate and proximate, and mediate and remote. Immediate material cooperation involves participating in the sinful act itself, not merely participating in an act that makes the sinful act possible (Koch 1933, 41). Engaging in immediate material cooperation without sin is rarely possible. Mediate material cooperation involves participating in an act that is secondary or subservient to the sinful act of another. *Proximate* and *remote* refer to the moral distance between the agent performing the sinful act and the individual who participates in the secondary or subservient act. In the case of proximate and mediate cooperation, the individual participates in an act that is secondary or subservient to the sinful act of another but is very closely connected to the sinful act of the other. Remote and mediate cooperation involves participating in an act that is secondary or subservient to the sinful act of another and is not closely connected to the sinful act (Davis 1936, 341–42).

Case Studies

The following cases touch on these points and illustrate the role of conscience in the decision making of Filipinos. They are heuristic of the complex interplay of cultural, religious, and socioeconomic values in the developing world.

CASE 1: Maternity Hospital is noted for its excellent ob-gyn residency program. Dr. Pablo is a consultant in this hospital. After Dr. Pablo's daughter graduates from medical school, Dr. Pablo encourages her to join Maternity Hospital's residency program. He assures her that she will be accepted. The program includes participation in performing a required number of tubal ligations. Dr. Pablo's daughter is not only a Catholic but a graduate of a Catholic university. Although the Philippines is a Roman Catholic country, not only is direct sterilization legal and widely performed in the non-Catholic hospitals, it is encouraged by the government.

ANALYSIS: Certainly this situation would pose moral problems for the believing and practicing Catholic physician. The situation may become complicated because of the pressure that may be applied by Dr. Pablo and her family generally. Given the difficulty in gaining admittance into a good residency program, the pressure may become even stronger. By Catholic standards, participation in tubal ligation constitutes immediate material cooperation and therefore is morally illicit. Dr. Pablo's daughter may claim that she would not intend the performance of the act. Yet she would in fact perform the vile act. At the very least, she is involved in immediate material cooperation in a forbidden act.

Therefore, in Catholic morality such participation is not permissible. Her action falls under the general maxim that no one is allowed to do an evil act intentionally, either as an end or as a means.

One would expect that the decision will depend on the strength of the daughter's Catholic moral convictions. One would not be surprised if she consults with a Catholic priest to ease her conscience. Eventually, she will face a serious conflict between her personal conscience and the official teaching of the Roman Catholic Church, which runs counter to the moral position of the government. Granting, however, that she chooses to accept the residency program, judging the subjective state of decision making would be difficult, given the complex factors that may influence her decision.

The conflicting moral positions of the Church and the government engender conflicts of conscience among young Filipino physicians and patients. They raise the question of what role physicians should play with regard to religious questions posed by patients. There will be a salience of religious moral concerns that is rare in the United States, except perhaps around the issue of abortion.

CASE 2: Manuela is scheduled for a hysterectomy because of cancer of the uterus. A resident who is to assist in the surgery discovers that Manuela is also two months pregnant. Manuela is not aware of her pregnancy; she has attributed all of her symptoms to her cancer. When the resident asks Dr. Garcia about informing Manuela, Dr. Garcia explains that he has intentionally not told Manuela of her pregnancy. He claims that telling her would unnecessarily depress her further.

ANALYSIS: Dr. Garcia's position is a classic example of conflicting norms of truth-telling, which arise from the demands of the Western bioethical standards of autonomy and beneficence. Dr. Garcia may not even attempt to balance the two principles before he makes the decision, however. His decision may come simply from his paternalistic moral sense about the right thing for the patient. Moreover, Dr. Garcia, in conformity with Roman Catholic doctrine, believes the procedure can be justified under the principle of double effect. The act is intended to remove cancer, which has a side effect of killing the unborn child. The resident, however, still may feel obliged to tell the truth to the patient. Because of his respect for the consultant, however, he may keep that desire to himself.

Again, one sees that the logic of Filipino bioethics is remarkably different from that of the West. Issues such as avoiding a direct abortion have salience, whereas concerns with consent and personal autonomy retreat into the background. In short, the two moral worlds have quite different understandings of what is morally relevant and how to approach and resolve moral controversies.

References

Davis, H., S.J. 1936. *Moral and Pastoral Theology, Volume I: Human Acts, Law, Sin, Virtue.* New York: Sheed and Ward.

Koch, A., D.D. 1933. *A Handbook of Moral Theology, Volume V.* St. Louis and London: B. Herder Book Co.

Honesty, Loyalty, and Cheating

Angeles Tan Alora

Among the challenges of framing a bioethics for the developing world are the ways in which apparently familiar moral concerns, such as honesty, may be radically recast by local circumstances. In the Philippines, honesty is understood in the context of personalism, which incorporates the concepts of *utang na loob* and *pakikisama*. Determination of what is beneficial is viewed in relation to advantages to the person, or the person's group or family, rather than in terms of society as a whole. Contextualized in this way, honesty is an issue of personalism rather than legalism. It is a matter of loyalty rather than an issue of integrity. Honest action is evaluated not so much in light of its impact on the entire society as in terms of its function in maintaining important personal relationships.

An "honest" person pays attention to personal relations within Filipino society. For instance, one does not steal from a person with whom one has a close relationship. House servants rarely steal from their masters. Yet an "honest" person may steal from an institution or the government because they are regarded as nonhuman entities and therefore of less concern. Filipinos commonly use company supplies for private needs, submit padded bills, or even evade taxes. The morality of stealing also is conceptualized in terms of what is stolen. Taking material, measurable goods would be wrong, whereas taking nonmaterial, less measurable goods would not. Stealing a sack of rice is wrong, but going home from work early or doing less than one's best is considered excusable. Although this attitude might work for the good of particular social groups, it has been criticized as a stumbling block to the development of social consciousness among the Filipino people.

Such a conception of honesty is manifested in medical education as well as in health care practice. For instance, cheating on classroom examinations or with regard to medical certificates is common. Rather than being condemned, such practices are rationalized as cultural norms, helping another person, or avoiding a greater evil. No doubt, a contributing factor is that those in authority often admit to having been dishonest while working toward their own position. For example, teachers often admit to their students that they cheated as students. A remark such as, "It is okay to cheat as long as I do not catch you" is common. Moreover, Filipinos know well that corruption in government is the norm.

Truth-telling is not always considered a virtue, and full disclosure often is regarded as a heinous vice. Telling someone that her dress is not pretty is impolite and unkind. When the information is bad news, one should kindly withhold the information or even tell a lie. Telling a lie to avoid hurting someone else is regarded as virtuous.

Case I: Cheating in Medical School

While taking undergraduate medical examinations, Mandaraya copies answers from his classmate's test. His slogan is "better cheat than repeat." When he is asked about this practice, he says that 90 percent of the medical students in his medical school cheat on examinations.

ANALYSIS: Medical students cheat on exams. Cheating occurs in different forms, including gaining access to test questions before exams, bringing notes to the examination, copying a classmate's answers, altering answers on returned papers, and so forth. Although most students regard these acts as wrong, they also consider them necessary to survive in the stressful and competitive world of medical school. They judge such dishonesty to be a lesser evil than failure.

Many cultural values are associated with classroom cheating. If a student fails, family pride and parental expectations are hurt. The high cost of another year in medical school burdens a family severely. It may even disrupt family harmony. Students allow others to copy because refusing goes against the value of caring and *pakikisama*. It might even be considered a lack of kindness toward a failing classmate.

Case II: The Child Born Dead

During delivery, Bagsak is dropped from the hands of a receiving intern and dies immediately. Her parents are informed that Bagsak was born dead.

ANALYSIS: Telling Bagsak's parents that Bagsak was born dead is dishonest. It is making a claim that one knows to be false. Yet a variety of considerations that are well-embedded in Filipino culture favor not informing the parents that their newborn was dropped. The harm has been done; telling the truth will not undo it. The parents do not need the information because no further treatment decision must be made for their child. Most important, telling the truth in this case would not be compassionate. The parents are likely to have an easier time accepting the fact that their child was born dead than the fact that their child was dropped. Why cause additional hurt when it is unnecessary?

Moreover, in the Philippines the likelihood of a civil action for recovery is small, and no distinction would be made on the part of many Filipinos between an injury resulting from natural causes and one resulting from human error. Why risk disrupting harmony between parent and physician or risk a lawsuit?

Again, the logic of Filipino decision making focuses on a view of well-being that is quite unlike that characteristic of Western bioethical reflections. Whereas in Western bioethics the emphasis would be on autonomy and truth-telling, in Filipino bioethical reflection, the emphasis is on harmony.

Case III: Dr. Sekreto's Secret

Pacencia has carcinoma of the womb. Dr. Sekreto tells her this diagnosis, and she becomes deeply depressed. He does not inform her that she also is pregnant because he is afraid that the knowledge would worsen her depression. She does not suspect that she is pregnant because she attributes the cessation of her menstrual periods and her swelling to the tumor. Dr. Sekreto decides to operate on Pacencia to remove the womb (thus, also to kill the fetus) without revealing the pregnancy to her.

ANALYSIS: In Western bioethics, the issue is simple. Pacencia has the right to decide what will be done to her body. To make such decisions, she needs correct and complete information. Pregnancy is vital information. The information may lead Pacencia to decide against surgery. Nevertheless, any information that will affect the decision may not be withheld. Thus, in Western bioethical terms Dr. Sekreto must tell Pacencia that she is pregnant.

In the East, however, physicians often make decisions concerning what should be done to the patient's body in the patient's best interests. In this case, Dr. Sekreto decides on behalf of Pacencia that the uterus and tumor must be removed, including the fetus. He does not regard informing her of her pregnancy as necessary. He, not Pacencia, must make the decision in this case. Dr. Sekreto also is concerned that telling Pacencia about the pregnancy would make her more depressed and therefore would cause harm. Hence, he uses his therapeutic privilege paternalistically to withhold the information. This attitude is expected of an authority figure within the Filipino culture.

Case IV: Should a Doctor Lie?

Botchok, a 24-year-old young man, suffers from end-stage renal disease and needs a kidney transplant. Botchok is the eldest son of Mr. and Mrs. Tabachoy. Two years ago he graduated from a Medical Technology course and immediately found a job. He has voluntarily used his earnings to support his sister

Tingting, a third-year Bachelor of Science in Education student. Mr. and Mrs. Tabachoy hold very high hopes for Botchok. Mr. and Mrs. Tabachoy know that they cannot afford a transplant for their son. They hope they can find a donor among their family members to save Botchok's life.

Within the family, only Tingting's tissue matches Botchok's. Tingting does not want to donate her kidney, however. She agreed to be tested because she did not want to disappoint Botchok or her parents. Now she is afraid of the operation and its consequences. Tingting's boyfriend Ugok warns her that losing a kidney would risk her capacity to have healthy pregnancies. Ugok also tells Tingting that his parents expect him to offer them grandchildren because he is the only child of the family. To avoid appearing ungrateful and being shamed in front of her family, Tingting requests that Dr. Laslas inform her family that her tissue does not match Botchok's.

ANALYSIS: In modern Western culture, donating a kidney is primarily a matter of charity, love, and generosity. No one is obliged to donate. In the Filipino culture, however, donation also is a family issue that entails familial allegiances. Refusing to donate to a family member is against the Filipino commitments to family support, *utang na loob,* and *pakikisama*. It can lead to serious family shame. At the same time, however, in this case refusing to donate shows respect for the authority of Tingting's future in-laws. The Filipino concern for *lusot* would suggest and support lying.

In the Philippines, the physician's response will depend on his or her relationships with individual members of the family. The more closely the physician is related to Mr. and Mrs. Tabachoy, the more likely he will encourage Tingting to donate. He may even volunteer to talk to Ugok to dispel him of his misconceptions concerning kidney donation and its effects on future pregnancies. On the other hand, if Dr. Laslas feels closer to Tingting, he is likely to defer to her request and provide her with *palusot,* an excuse.

Case V: Personal Loyalty versus Professional Integrity

Direk, a 52-year-old internist, is the director of a 150-bed hospital. His responsibilities include approving drugs for purchase by the hospital pharmacy. Kabayan, a townmate and former medical school classmate who dropped out of medical school and formed a drug company, approaches Direk to purchase antibiotics from the Kabayan Drug Company.

When Direk and Kabayan were students, they were like brothers. Kabayan even lent money to Direk to assist in paying his tuition. Direk notes, however, that the prices of Kabayan's drugs are 30–40 percent higher than other bidders'. Direk also knows that Kabayan's company was banned a couple of years ago because his drugs caused untoward side effects, such as rashes and urticaria. Kabayan assures Direk that his products have been retested and improved. He explains that this is why the current prices of his drugs are higher.

ANALYSIS: There is a distinct tension between Direk's professional responsibilities and his personal relationship. On one hand, he ought to show loyalty to the hospital—a legal but nonhuman entity; on the other hand, he must maintain his personal loyalty to his friend. Within the Filipino culture, this tension is very real and very difficult.

As a hospital director, Direk owes loyalty to his institution. If he approves the purchase of Kabayan's products, the hospital will lose financially because of the higher prices. In addition, the previous incidence of side effects places the hospital's patients at potential risk of harm from those drugs, in spite of Kabayan's assurance that the problem has been solved. Disregarding a long-standing personal relationship, however, is unthinkable within Filipino culture. If Direk refuses to purchase drugs from Kabayan, he will be branded as *walang utang na loob* (no debt of gratitude)—an ingrate. This decision may even damage his family's name and social standing. His obligations to Kabayan have widely acknowledged standing.

Although such a decision would have real costs to the impersonal institution (the hospital) as well as to identifiable persons (i.e., patients), Direk probably would choose personal loyalty over professional integrity. Filipino culture demands it. An appreciation of appropriate moral action sustains a set of important moral commitments. All else being equal, obligations of gratitude trump abstract moral commitments. Indeed, moral obligations to institutions rather than human beings (to whom one has a moral debt of gratitude) bear the burden of proof. That is, obligations to human beings trump obligations to institutions unless the latter can be shown to have a very clear and convincing claim. The moral claims of persons do not simply outweigh contrary claims by institutions; the latter often bear the *onus probandi*.

The result is a moral world that is quite different from the one that obtains in most western European and North American cultures. The latter presume that morality is an anonymous project that is devoid of particular claims generated out of special past relationships of obligation or debt that can justify lying and cheating. Whereas the western European/North American moral culture considers such lying and cheating worthy of blame and morally corruptive, the moral culture of the Philippines finds the very opposite. The moral disarticulation, fragmentation, and anomie of the West is likely to be the result of its misguided emphasis on morality as an anonymous project embedded in a view from nowhere. The Philippines considers the collapse of Western familial relationships to be a result of the failure to recognize special personal obligations. The result is a true conflict of moralities and bioethics. There is a conflict not just of particular obligations but regarding the very sense or meaning of morality.

Here as elsewhere, one finds an important difference between the standard American version of bioethics and that of the Philippines and much of the developing world. They have radically different understandings of the character of the moral point of view. They do not simply give different orderings to important moral values or principles. They differ with respect to whether the moral point of view is anonymous and disinterested or highly personalistic and agent-relative in reflecting local (e.g., familial and personal) debts and relationships.

Philanthropy and Nepotism

Angelica Francisco

To juxtapose philanthropy with nepotism in health care would seem to emphasize the inappropriateness of such a combination. In the Filipino culture of contradictions (from the perspective of western European / North American morality), however, these two concepts are complementary. In fact, they form a continuum. Defined in the Christian context, which applies to approximately 85 percent of the Filipino population, philanthropy is the "expression of an unlimited, freely given, sacrificial love that was not dependent on the worthiness of its object" (Amundsen 1995). Therefore, assistance is extended to people in need regardless of other considerations. Nepotism, on the other hand, discriminates and gives preference to one's relatives. Hence, there is a continuum from the objective and general in philanthropy to the subjective and particular in nepotism.

What is common to philanthropy and nepotism is that each provides means by which individuals can avail themselves of the resources in society. When resources are scarce, the scramble for what is available becomes highly competitive. In such circumstances, how are decisions made regarding who shall receive which resources, and how much? What is the Filipino concept of justice? How do Filipinos decide what is owed to their fellows? What are the background expectations behind health care resource decision making?

To answer these questions, one must study Filipinos in the social context in which they live, become ill, seek health care, and provide medical services. Two levels of relationships are distinguished on the basis of *ibang-tao* (the outgroup) and *hindi ibang-tao* (the in-group) (Miranda 1995). Furthermore, the Filipino culture refers to three basic spheres of interaction: *kami,* the innermost circle, the in-group, commonly made up of the nuclear family and occasionally very close friends; *tayo,* the middle circle, formed by acquaintances and friendly strangers; and *sila,* the outer circle, formed by "unfriendly" strangers. These distinctions largely reflect how important the family is to Filipinos. Besides being the basic unit of social structure, the family is regarded as an important value in itself. It is intrinsically valuable; it is the source of values. Familial values have *prima facie* precedence over most other values. Moral choices have a family-regarding character. The Filipino family is the individual's ever-reliable—if not inexhaustible—source of spiritual, material, and medical support.

Never have hierarchical distinctions been more strongly emphasized than in the Filipino family, especially among *Tagalog*-speaking Christians. Siblings refer to each other according to a rank-ordering: The eldest son is called *"kuya"*; next is *"diku,"* then *"sangko"* and *"siko."* The equivalent rankings for daughters are *"ate," "ditse," "sanse,"* and *"dete."* Inherent in this hierarchy is the respect that the younger siblings should render to their elders. In exchange, these distinctions also emphasize the duty and obligation of the older children to look after the welfare of the younger ones. From this ranking, one also can infer the large size of the traditional Filipino family (often 8–10 children). The expectation that older children will share in the responsibility of rearing the younger ones physically and financially is a cultural derivative from a basically agricultural economy.

Similarly, the Filipino concept of justice finds parallels in the organization of and relationships within the family. A popular phrase that refers to distribution of goods is *hating-kapatid* (literally, sharing-by-siblings). This term refers to the act of one dividing and the other having first choice regarding the preferred portion. Variations include behaviors whereby one forgoes his or her share in favor of whoever needs it more. Inherent in these cases is the recognition that actual divisions cannot produce exact equality.

The acceptance of social inequality may derive from the organization of precolonial tribal groups. The historical literature cites the inherent inequality in the class distinctions in precolonial Filipino communities, the *baranggay* (Gorospe 1976), where each class was entitled to different rights and privileges. These classes included the *marharlika* (the ruling class), the *aliping-malaya* (freed slaves), and the *aliping saguiguilid* (bonded slaves). The rights and privileges enjoyed by the upper class demand corresponding responsibilities, however. The emphasis is on the duty of the privileged class to look after the welfare of the lower classes. Members of the privileged class are entitled to respect and loyalty as long as they fulfill their obligations to the rest of the community.

In the context of this web of Filipino family and community loyalties, how does nepotism extend to philanthropy? This extremely family-centered moral consciousness has been criticized as the root cause of obstacles that impede the development of a nation-oriented moral consciousness (Gorospe 1976). In fact, these commitments have institutionalized a widespread phenomenon in Filipino society, euphemistically termed *Kamag-anak, Inc.* ("Relatives, Inc."). In governmental offices, this practice means that Filipinos who gain office begin by hiring their own relatives to fill available positions. These practices, as well as others, may be advanced as grounds for criticizing the Filipino moral point of view. Indeed, different moral geographies have different moral costs and benefits. A sternly anonymous moral point of view places the burden of proof on moral choices that are directed to personal moral relationships and debts. From this perspective, one will tend to avoid nepotism, but one will also tend to undercut familial structures that depend at least in part on the reinforcement of familial bonds through the reciprocal discharge of familial debts.

All virtues may become vices if carried to extremes. Moreover, what might appear to be a vice to Western moralists may appear morally neutral, if not morally praiseworthy, in the Filipino moral understanding. An example is nepotism. Although nepotism usually is considered to be a vice, at the other end of the spectrum it also may have positive value. In a society in which resources are scarce, the presence of philanthropy expressed through impartial institutions is rare, and anonymous moral responses are not enough to fulfill the prevailing needs of the population. Where formal institutions of philanthropy fail, the family must step in to fill the gap. More significantly, the web of familial moral obligations sustains a moral life-world that often is nonexistent in the culture of North America. Nepotism is integral to a province of moral experience.

These different domains of moral experience direct philanthropic action in very different ways. In each domain we must ask, Whom do we help? How much and what kind of help do we extend? In the circle of relationships, the conditions within the *kami* are taken to be absolute and all-encompassing. In contrast to questions raised about families in the West (Nelson and Nelson 1995), no limits are set on the care the family owes its own, nor are there limits on the potential sacrifices of individual members. The only question is, What is needed? Filipinos take for granted that efforts will be made to meet this need regardless of the cost. Outside of *kami*, in *tayo*, limits are clearly laid down. The first question is, *Kaanu-ano ko ba siya?* ("How am I related to him?") Once a kinship is established, help might be extended, depending on the obligations established, the kind and amount of help needed, and how much one is willing or able to spare.

In *sila*, no kinship is established, nor is there the recognized duty or obligation to help. This is not to say that there is general social apathy within this sphere. At this level, one may offer charity or assistance because it is perceived to be the right thing to do. For example, the preponderance of mendicants who refuse to earn a living in other ways because they earn more by begging attests to this practice of what some Filipinos refer to as "misguided" philanthropy.

Aside from material wealth, which is in short supply, other forms of assistance often are extended. In the Filipino culture, the spirit of *bayanihan* ("being one with the community") often is exemplified through sharing of knowledge, skill, time, and sometimes even labor. In the health care profession, sharing of knowledge and skills is common in the conduct of medical missions. Any social function that doctors attend often becomes an extension of their clinic.

Although philanthropy seems to be inherent in medical care, the complex relationships arising from the society in which the Filipino doctor moves has made it an inherent part of medical practice. Indeed, a subclassification of patients for clinicians are NCs ("no-charges").

In summary, although nepotism has its critics, where individual needs are not met by other institutions, the family must assume the burden of taking care of its own. This form of nepotism is so common as to be the norm. Seeking help through relatives functions as a way of equalizing the odds in one's favor, of gaining access to the limited resources that public funds have made available. In the community, the limits of obligations set by relationships are sufficiently fluid that in most circumstances common grounds are established for assistance and cooperation. At stake are fundamentally different understandings of the project of morality.

CASE: St. Cosmas Tuberculosis Clinic provides free treatment to approximately 500 indigent tuberculosis (TB) patients. Funds have been progressively more difficult to acquire in spite of numerous requests to various charitable institutions and foundations. The staff decides to employ Alice Tan, a new medical graduate who has not yet passed the medical boards. Alice is the daughter of Lucas Tan, chairman of several foundations. Previously, none of Mr. Tan's foundations have been directly involved in health care delivery. After two months, St. Cosmas TB Clinic receives a foundation educational grant of 2 million pesos.

ANALYSIS: In this instance, an act of philanthropy is motivated by very personal considerations. The act of beneficence is justified not by an appeal to a disinterested moral view from nowhere but in terms of a very particular, content-rich, family-oriented view from somewhere. The fabric of moral assumptions and the assessment of which moral considerations trump other factors establish a moral framework that is very different from the framework that is officially endorsed in the West. This is not the standard American bioethical world of principles, casuistry, and balancing claims. The principles are substantially different, the framing of the casuistry assumes a different set of cardinal moral structures, and moral claims are weighed in very differently calibrated balances.

References

Amundsen, D. 1995. Early Christianity. In *Encyclopedia of Bioethics*, vol. 3, edited by W. T. Reich. New York: Simon & Schuster, 1519.

Gorospe, V. 1976. Sources of Filipino Moral Consciousness. In *Morality, Religion and the Filipino: Essays in Honor of Vitaliano R. Gorospe, S.J.*, edited by R. B. Javellana, S.J. Quezon City, The Philippines: Ateneo de Manila University Press, 1–23.

Miranda, D. 1995. *Buting Pinoy: Probe Essays on Value as Filipino*. Manila: Divine Word Publications.

Nelson, H., and J. Nelson. 1995. Family. In *Encyclopedia of Bioethics*, vol. 2, edited by W. T. Reich. New York: Simon & Schuster, 801–08.

PART IV

Facing Hard Choices

Ethical Issues in the Pediatric Intensive Care Unit

Angeles Tan Alora and Mary Jean Villareal-Guno

Pediatric intensive care units (PICUs) and neonatal intensive care units (NICUs) were established in the Philippines in the 1980s. At the University of Santo Tomas' private Catholic hospital, the PICU was established in July 1987. It was created with a generous donation from a group of medical alumni for the dual purpose of improving health care delivery to critically ill children and providing future medical professionals with training in pediatric intensive care.

The hospital is made up of two separate divisions: the clinical and the private. The clinical division serves as the teaching hospital for the medical school and provides affordable, quality medical care for indigent patients by charging only at cost for procedures, medications, supplies, laboratory services, and equipment. Professional fees, room charges, and meals are provided free of charge. The private division partially subsidizes the cost of operating the clinical division. In the private division, wealthy patients pay a premium for quicker access to health care, expensive treatments, and private rooms. Such cost shifting allows the hospital to continue its charitable work.

The three-bed PICU was built in the clinical division to serve indigent patients. Families who can afford to pay are encouraged to make donations to sustain the unit. Despite minimal charges, however, many indigent families still are unable to afford the cost of PICU care. Yet when parents are presented with life-and-death decisions between providing or withholding life-sustaining care or between using ordinary and extraordinary means of sustaining life, they usually ask the physicians to "do everything for the child." Their overall concern, as well as their desire to provide their children with the best possible care, reflects the value Filipinos place on children. It reflects the central Filipino value of family-centeredness (*pagpapahalaga sa pamilya*). The family is the highest value in Filipino culture; it functions as the core of all social and economic activity. Closeness and solidarity mark the Filipino family, and children are always considered a blessing.

At times, however, interpreting what "everything" or "all" means is difficult. Although the patient's family often desires every possible advantage that technology can offer, in hope of a miracle, society often interprets "everything" to imply reasonable efforts that reflect a manifestation of concern or care for the patient. Physicians, on the other hand, typically understand such a call as a request for any action that may save life, allow the patient to survive longer, or relieve suffering.

In any case, the qualifying phrase "that helps the patient" should be added to "everything." Futile measures that unnecessarily prolong the dying process and waste resources should be avoided. Ill children are considered gifts from God, sources of family strength and possible good luck, or indications of coming rewards for the family. In caring for these children, physicians tend to look toward the probabilities of survival rather than the expected quality of life of the children.

Families often promise to exhaust all private resources and borrow funds to pay for additional care. Even in the case of terminally ill patients who are close to death, whose treatment is futile and burdensome to the family, parents typically are hesitant to withdraw care. The concern is that withholding life support measures, even when doing so is ethically justifiable, constitutes child abandonment and a failure to fulfill parental obligations.

This feeling reflects the Filipino attitude of *bahala na*. Such an attitude signifies a willingness to take chances and risks no matter what difficulties and problems the future will entail. It reflects an almost superstitious belief or blind faith in fate, as escape from decision making and social responsibility. It also is a manifestation of trust in God (Gorospe 1988), or of giving the whole of one's life to God. When parents confront critical or stressful situations, they hope that a miracle will transpire, that their child will improve, and that God will take care of everything.

The *bahala na* attitude is a fatalistic resignation that represents a withdrawal from engagement or crisis or a shrinking away from responsibility. *Bahala na* also can engender a false sense of security with God as a sort of personal insurance. Days may pass during which hospital bills remain unsettled and the family is unable to purchase needed medication, until the child eventually dies from the medical condition. In a country in which almost all of the cost of medical care is shouldered by the family, this attitude raises financial and ethical problems (Andres 1988; Miranda 1992).

Another important ethical issue in pediatrics is whether children ought to be involved in decisions regarding their own health care. The strong sense of family solidarity in the Philippines means that decisions usually are made as a group, with the head of the family having the final word. Authoritarianism is a primary value in Filipino culture, resulting from the close family kinship of the Filipino and the ways in which respect for parents is strongly emphasized (Gorospe 1988). Patterns of interdependence are fostered by the traditional Filipino family, with emphasis on respect for parents as authority figures. In the process of disclosing information and seeking treatment decisions, health care professionals rarely involve the affected child. The head of the family is the ultimate decision maker. Teenagers and young adults do not mind the lack of personal consultation because they rely on their families for support, care, and concern.

The financial difficulties of maintaining a PICU and the 50 percent survival rate of admitted patients have resulted in a hospital policy that gives priority (if not exclusive admission privileges) to acutely ill patients for whom ventilator support offers a high probability of success. Ancillary diagnostic workups are limited to the most essential tests. Moreover, discussing the cost of PICU care with the family prior to admission is strongly encouraged. For families who would be overburdened by the probable expenses, government institutions are immediately approached for resources.

This system raises questions, however, regarding who ought to be regarded as in authority to determine whether there is great or little hope of survival. Predicting survival is even more difficult in pediatric practice, compared to such prediction for adults, because criteria have not been clearly set and available studies are often wanting. Ethical issues shroud the extension of PICU care for patients where the provision of intensive treatment would merely prolong the agony of dying or would be ineffective in ameliorating an infant's life-threatening condition. Even the criteria for brain-death determination raise serious questions when applied to children (Barclay 1981). Consequently, the medical staff at the University of Santo Tomas hospital has had to rely primarily on clinical judgment in predicting the probability of survival.

Particularly difficult ethical questions for pediatric care include concerns with patient autonomy, shared decision making, and the dilemma of balancing harms and benefits in pediatric intensive care. Such concerns are further complicated in cases that involve minors and in which the highly valued traditions of family privacy and parental authority are at issue (American Academy of Pediatrics and American College of Emergency Physicians 1989).

CASE 1: C. B., a six-month-old female, was admitted for ventilator support in the PICU with a diagnosis of bacterial meningitis, hypoxic encephalopathy, aspiration pneumonia, and recent cardiac arrest. She was comatose and apneic, with absent reflexes. The medical team felt the prognosis was very poor and discussed with the family the concept of brain death. The parents insisted that all medical support be given at any cost because this child was precious, the youngest of three children. On the fourth hospital day, C. B. died. The family had an unsettled hospital bill of P7,000.00.

ANALYSIS: There is no generally accepted definition of brain death in a neonate. As a result, the medical team determines when the individual is dead.

This determination is affected by their individual competence and even their subjective feelings and evaluations of the patient's situation. Through constant dialogue, health care providers attempt to allow time for the family to grasp the painful reality of death and emotionally to prepare to accept the death of their child. In the meantime, life support measures are sustained, and bills accumulate. Because Filipinos have limited access to insurance or to church or government subsidies, the nuclear and extended family is expected to shoulder the bills. When the family is unable to pay for care, whose burden is it? Private hospitals typically are left to assume the financial burden. If such a circumstance happens in this and similar cases, continued losses could lead to the closure of hospital units or the entire hospital or render the institution unable to provide affordable quality medical care to indigent individuals, including those with greater chances of survival.

CASE 2: Baby S. was born prematurely, at 25 weeks gestational age, to a 21-year-old unwed mother who had taken multiple abortifacients. At birth, the baby was limp, with no spontaneous respiration, poor cardiac activity, and no response to stimuli. Manual respiration, antibiotics, and hydration were initiated. In this private, tertiary-care center, the age of viability in the NICU is 28–30 weeks gestational age. The mother requested that the physician do whatever was possible but stated that she could not sustain the expenses of the NICU, which would amount to approximately P10,000 per day for equipment and medication. After 48 hours, the baby went into cardiac arrest. No aggressive resuscitative efforts were undertaken, and she died.

ANALYSIS: This case raises a cluster of related issues. Given that the likelihood of success is poor, may the staff withhold mechanical ventilator and other life-support measures without informing the mother? Should the fact that the mother is unwed affect treatment decisions? If aggressive support measures are pursued in the care of this baby, who should carry the burden of cost? On another level, how will the NICU improve its age of viability if attempts to sustain such infants are not undertaken?

In this particular case, the child received the care and respect due a human being (a warm environment, manual ventilation, hydration, and antibiotics) (see McCormick 1984). This treatment was not overly aggressive, however; nature was allowed to take its course. Constant dialogue should be carried out with parents to keep them informed about the situation and the most probable outcomes. Counseling should be made available to parents to help them work through the emotional impact of the child's death. Any "do not resuscitate" order should be discussed in detail in advance, and all pertinent decisions should be recorded in the chart (Brody and Engelhardt 1987; Engelhardt and Rie 1986).

CASE 3: J. L., a four-year-old male, was admitted to the PICU for ventilator support with a diagnosis of ventricular septal defect, not in failure, broncho-pneumonia, and status asthmaticus. The medical team wanted to give him maximal support because they felt the present crisis could be reversed. The family agreed with the team but could not purchase all of the medications required. Available PICU funds for indigent patients and other social services funds had been exhausted, and the unsettled hospital bills accumulated to P60,000. No funds were available for further PICU care, much less for corrective surgical intervention. J. L. died after 20 days.

ANALYSIS: Decisions regarding which patients are to receive life-prolonging measures are different in the Philippines than they are in the United States. In the United States, Baby Doe laws mandate initial aggressive treatment. In the Philippines, however, limited resources and acceptance of God's will may mandate initial withholding of aggressive measures. The fear of societal disapproval and interpretation of such actions as patient abandonment may lead, however, to new policies to avoid over- and undertreating such children.

This case typifies the hospital situation in the Philippines. Because poor families have no money, they generally fail to seek help during the early course of an illness and simply hope that the child will improve. They do not realize that early intervention could prevent the development of a serious situation that could generate greater expenses. Patients often are brought in when they are very sick or dying, when the medical team and the family have limited resources available to reverse such critical situations. In this case, the medical staff believed that the probability of success was high and the prognosis was good. Eventually, however, resources were depleted, and the patient died without receiving effective care.

In short, a cluster of moral and cultural expectations move parents to expend large sums of money on the treatment of imperiled newborns even when there is little likelihood of conveying a benefit. The technological imperative has a special cultural urgency, leading to the paradox that scarce medical resources are invested disproportionately in high-cost, high-intensity pediatric care while routine pediatric care often is unavailable because of limited medical and financial resources.

References

Andres, T. D. 1988. *Understanding Filipino Values*. Manila: New Day Publishing.

American Academy of Pediatrics and American College of Emergency Physicians. 1989. *Advanced Pediatric Life Support*. Elk Grove, Ill.: American Academy of Pediatrics; Dallas: American College of Emergency Physicians.

Barclay, W. R. 1981. Guidelines of the determination of death. *Journal of the American Medical Association* 246(19): 2194.

Brody, B., and H. T. Engelhardt. 1987. *Bioethics: Readings and Cases*. Englewood Cliffs, N.J.: Prentice Hall.

Engelhardt, H. T., and M. Rie. 1986. Intensive care units, scarce resources, and conflicting principles of justice. *Journal of the American Medical Association* 255(9): 1159–64.

Gorospe, V. 1988. *Filipino Values Revisited*. Manila: National Book Store.

McCormick, R. 1984. *Health and Medicine in the Catholic Tradition*. New York: Crossroads.

Miranda, D. M. 1992. *Buting Pinoy*. Manila: Divine Word Publications.

AIDS in the Developing World: The Case of the Philippines

Josephine M. Lumitao

AIDS has produced one of the most serious health crises of our time. Compelling and tragic stories of failures by health workers to provide health care services, tell the truth, or maintain confidentiality and privacy are increasing. The number of symposia and papers that deal with ethical problems linked to AIDS make clear that these problems are important and pressing, and that they are evolving rapidly and have no easy solutions. Caring for the increasing number of AIDS patients and creating policies to prevent the spread of the disease is a challenge to every physician who tries to practice ethically. In the developing world, the AIDS epidemic tends to have a large number of heterosexual transmissions. Thus, the disease cannot be easily closeted to a particular portion of society, as often occurs in developed countries.

The first AIDS case in the Philippines was reported in 1984. As of June 1997, the AIDS registry of the Department of Health had identified a total of 916 seropositives. Full-blown AIDS had been found in 310 patients; 159 had died. Males outnumbered females, and heterosexual contact was considered the primary mode of transmission (see Table 1, p. 151). In spite of the abundant resources poured into research to discover a therapeutic agent for AIDS, the disease remains lethal, and medications discovered may only prolong survival and make life more comfortable.

The impact of AIDS on developed countries, with their vast resources, has been tremendous (Mertz, Sushinsky, and Vao Schüklenk 1996; Boisaubin 1991; Council for Ethical and Judicial Affairs 1988). The effect of AIDS on developing countries, with their economic constraints and social problems, may reach such an unquantifiable magnitude that local statistics may not be credible.

Bioethical issues related to AIDS—such as confidentiality, truth-telling, providing health care to individual patients, and protection of others / community—assume different circumstantial features in the context of Filipino culture. The pivotal role of the family in all aspects of the individual's life affects the individual's health care issues, confidentiality, and truth-telling. Socioeconomic factors and allocation of health care resources affect efforts to prevent the spread of infection. This essay analyzes the complex interplay of these factors to portray unique bioethical issues that AIDS creates in developing countries in general and the Philippines in particular.

Cultural and Socioeconomic Factors

The Filipino culture puts a great deal of emphasis on the family's central role in the individual's life. Filipinos make decisions and perform actions based not only on their own personal and individual benefit but on the family's welfare as well. The family encroaches into every aspect of individual life, including even the choice of a career or a marriage partner, as well as decisions in health care. Filipinos are expected to protect and uphold the family name. The success and awards an individual receives reflect on his or her parents' and family's prestige. The scandal and wrongdoing a Filipino commits will consequently cause a grave injury and dishonor to his or her family.

The diagnosis of AIDS, with its proven, specific methods of infection, carries a social and moral stigma with which most Filipino families would abhor to be associated. Consequently, AIDS patients do not want their families to know their diagnosis. With any other disease, patients would willingly play the role of a sick family member and let the family take over. Not so with AIDS. Some patients request that their diagnosis be changed to another, less stigmatizing disease (such as hepatitis) with similar medical implications to escape the discrimination and ostracism associated with this disease (Alora 1992; Ross 1989).

Another factor contributing to such requests is the very poor (almost zero) observance of confidentiality. Filipinos automatically presume that everyone has the right to information just because they happen to be members of the patient's family (even if only a very distant relative). This lack of confidentiality is present even among health workers and hospital personnel; as a result, voluntary testing for AIDS does not receive popular support. Everyone will know if someone is HIV-positive, and this knowledge would result in discrimination and grave scandal not only for the individual but for his or her family as well. The discrimination and ostracism encountered by AIDS patients who have come out in the open is a stumbling block to proper care and counseling of these patients and tracing of their sexual contacts. They then continue to spread the infection. Because of this discrimination and the stigma the disease would cause to families, AIDS patients who are dying are denied their last wish to spend their last moments with their loved ones.

The poor practice of universal precautions against HIV infection also plays an unrecognized but significant role in the spread of infection. Because of financial constraints, gloves, needles, and syringes are not disposable; they are re-used. Although these medical implements are sterilized, standards of sterilization vary from hospital to hospital. Wearing of goggles and the use of other barrier protections that serve as protective devices is not standard practice while attending to injured patients or during surgery. The HIV test is expensive. Many blood banks do not test their blood and blood products for HIV because of the expense involved. Consequently, patients pay for blood that is not tested and may be HIV-positive. Lack of education concerning the importance of this universal precaution, force of habit, and a personalistic approach to patients contribute to the spread of infection.

Because the Philippines is a developing country in dire socioeconomic straits, it has its share of prostitution; some observers claim that it is a major factor in the spread of infection. Prostitution formerly was localized at specific regions (e.g., the sites of U.S. military bases and the Red Light District in Manila), where tracking down and following up the health condition and HIV status of these sex workers was done on a regular basis. The dismantling of U.S. bases resulted in the dispersal of these sex workers to different parts of the country, where follow-up became difficult, if not impossible. The drive against the Red Light District in Manila resulted in a cleaner image but widely disseminated prostitutes who could be HIV-positive and spreading infection. Filipino males' penchant for peer-group *barkada*, drinking sprees, and womanizing remains a large factor in the continued spread of HIV infection. The controversy over the use of condoms, which the Roman Catholic Church has condemned, paradoxically may have had some impact on diminishing chances of infection by encouraging their use (Ashley and O'Rourke 1989).

The increasing number of overseas workers may be another potential source of infection that contributes to HIV cases in the country. HIV testing is required for persons leaving the country but not for those entering the country. This practice seems to be discriminatory against Filipinos because it protects other countries from HIV-positive individuals but leaves the Philippines open to possible HIV seropositives who are liable to spread the disease.

Bioethical Issues

There are two sets of issues involved in AIDS: those related to health care for the individual patient and those related to the protection of others. Measures that address care for the individual often protect society as well.

Because a patient with AIDS could harm and even kill others, should he or she transmit the disease, contacts must be protected. Sources of infection can be identified by testing, and contacts can be protected by informing them of positive results. This procedure is easier said than done, however. Sources of infection are difficult to identify because they do not come for testing out of fear of discrimination arising from a positive result. In the few instances when people are voluntarily tested and turn out to be positive, many refuse to reveal their sexual contacts, especially their spouses, because of family condemnation and dishonor. Frequently, identification of sources of infection is a problem because of limited testing procedures related to the expense involved.

Many people believe that society has a duty to provide care to every person, with or without AIDS. In providing health care, society has to make choices between AIDS and other health concerns. Similarly, it has to choose among prevention, cure, and symptomatic treatment. There will always be the temptation to maximize health outcomes in all ways; in a country whose health budget allotment is only 2.8 percent, however, emphasis on low-cost, high-yield schemes (preventive, educational campaigns) may be all that the budget allows (see, e.g., Dwyer 1994).

Treatment of an AIDS patient in a developing country can involve an increased risk of acquiring the HIV virus. In the developing world, the question of whether a physician may refuse to treat a patient with AIDS has special force because full protection (e.g., goggles) may not be available to protect physicians and nurses who are involved in care. Moreover, if a physician accepts an AIDS patient, other patients may not want to avail themselves of the physician's services. A private physician might wish to refuse AIDS patients because of personal risk or the risk of diminished profits. The virtues of integrity, compassion, and solidarity mandate that because of the physician's voluntary commitment to the profession, the physician should undertake the care of AIDS patients. If the physician declines to do so, he or she falls short of a standard of practice that is implicit in his or her moral and professional commitment. Nevertheless, no one can condemn a physician who refuses to treat AIDS patients. Patients who are treated by unwilling doctors may suffer, and physicians who treat AIDS patients may be exposed to levels of risk that do not confront physicians in the developed world (Zuger and Miles 1988; Steinbrook et al. 1985).

There are two situations in which the individual physician may not refuse and has a specific duty to provide care: when the physician is an immediate agent of society and when he or she has voluntarily entered into the physician/patient contract. In the Philippines, there are distressing stories of HIV-positive patients who have been turned away even from government hospitals. Technological deficiencies resulting from economic factors and lack of education about universal precautions are some of the causes for such behavior. A certain government hospital has designated one wing for AIDS patients where they can register and receive appropriate care.

Terminally ill AIDS patients need to be told the truth. AIDS is one specific disease for which the patient may personally ask for the diagnosis and request confidentiality, even from the close family. This policy is understandable because of the hurt, disharmony, recrimination, scandal, and stigma that follow disclosure. The health care provider must accept this unpleasant task as part of his or her responsibility and learn the personal skills of conveying information and caring for the patient nonjudgmentally and with compassion and respect. Counseling for the patient to help cope with the disease is highly recommended.

The mean survival of AIDS patients after hospitalization for opportunistic infection in the Philippines, even with optimal treatment, is reported to be less than eight months. In the absence of expensive treatment that generally is unavailable in the developing world, patients die, no matter what level of care is provided.

Decisions to provide or withdraw treatment are based on futility or allocation of scarce resources. A decision to withdraw treatment because it is useless is based on futility. A decision to withdraw treatment because someone else can make better use of the resources necessary to provide such treatment is based on the allocation of scarce resources for rationing purposes. Whatever the basis, the decision must be made by the patient. The patient may have values that would make "futile" treatment worthwhile. The patient may want time to make peace, say good-bye to a loved one, or help a loved one accept his or her death.

Because of financial constraints, many Filipino HIV-positive patients forgo treatment so that whatever resources are left may be used by their family and loved ones for a better future. Such a decision should not be condemned as suicidal but seen as part of the cultural trait of fatalism and ever-present concern for one's family welfare.

Illustrative Cases

CASE 1: A 32-year-old prostitute has AIDS. She lives with her mother and two-year-old daughter in a rented apartment. Her weakness and emaciation have prevented her from working for the past month, so living expenses are covered by her mother's P8500/month salary as a telephone operator and her own savings of approximately P500,000. She has no other financial resources.

New antiviral therapy that promises to prolong and improve the quality of the patient's life costs P33,000/month; she will need these drugs for the rest of her life. In addition, she would need drugs to prevent and control the complications of AIDS. Ultimately, the patient will die. The government program for AIDS does not include the new antiviral drugs. The pharmaceutical company subsidizes individual cases for six months.

A Catholic by birth, the patient has neither gone to church regularly nor received the sacraments for the past eight years. Though estranged in practice from her Roman Catholic roots, she recognizes her duties to her daughter to be fully in accord with Filipino moral commitments. She chooses the government program and saves the money for her daughter's education.

ANALYSIS: This case illustrates the tension between competing goods for the patient's savings; the money could be used for antiviral therapy to prolong her life or reserved to raise and educate her daughter.

The patient's decision to forgo life-prolonging treatment in favor of her family is perfectly understandable from the Filipino point of view. She knows she has a terminal condition, and the stigma of her disease—incurred as an occupational hazard—will be erased and redeemed by the sacrifice of giving up treatment for the sake of her daughter's livelihood and education.

CASE 2: C. S. is a 40-year-old nurse who returns to the Philippines with AIDS. She requests that a physician help monitor her disease; she is on an AZT protocol, but she insists on strict confidentiality.

C. S. knows the hysteria that occurs when some Filipinos know a patient has AIDS. She specifically cites the case of a physician who went on vacation to avoid delivering a child for a pregnant patient with AIDS and the case of a pathologist who refused to do an autopsy on an AIDS patient who also was refused burial at the local cemetery. C. S. worries about how her family will react and how much shame she may bring to the family name. She hopes to spend her remaining time with her husband and two children. She needs their support, love, and care. As a nurse, she knows how AIDS is transmitted and will take all necessary precautions. She will inform everyone that she has hepatitis B. She threatens to go back to the United States to die rather than let her family know.

ANALYSIS: This case illustrates the important issue of confidentiality with AIDS patients. C. S.'s request that her family not be told of her diagnosis can be understood as resulting from fear of condemnation, discrimination, and ostracism of her family at the time she needs them most. Her request that her diagnosis be changed to hepatitis B is an effort to have a diagnosis that is more acceptable to her family. Hepatitis B is relatively common in the Philippines; it has similar medical implications in terms of avoiding intimate contact, but it does not have the moral and social stigma associated with AIDS.

The health care provider must try to convince C. S. that this ruse might not be successful in protecting her husband from exposure. As C. S. nears death, making her peace can be possible only by telling the truth. This situation presents a conflict between maintaining confidence and breaking confidentiality, between keeping the patient-physician relationship of trust, compassion, and maintaining social harmony and protecting innocent third parties from harm. C. S. should be convinced that if she really loves her family, she should tell the truth to prevent harming them.

CASE 3: G. H., a 45-year-old married male executive, tested positive for HIV. He apparently acquired the infection during a trip abroad. He requests that no report be filed and that his family not be told because the knowledge would be emotionally shattering for them.

ANALYSIS: This case is similar to Case 2, in that G. H. fears the emotional burden of the information for his family. His request not to tell his family is understandable because of his fear of the recriminations that would result from such disclosure. Yet his wife should be informed because she is at risk. If she is told, however, safeguarding confidentiality becomes next to impossible. Torn between protecting the family name and seeking emotional support from other family members, the wife is likely to tell a sister, a close friend, or her mother. Soon, extended family members will know. Even maids, drivers, and other household help will talk about it. The agents of disclosure multiply.

Many Filipinos who are caught in such situations seek radical solutions, such as going abroad for treatment if they can afford it or forgoing treatment if they cannot.

Conclusion

In the developing world, AIDS creates specific bioethical issues related to confidentiality, limited treatment options, special construals of provision of care for the patient, and protection of others/society. The role of the family as the decision maker, the fear of moral and social stigma, and discrimination affect how one approaches confidentiality, as well as accurate reporting of cases. Financial constraints create potential new sources of infection because of recycling of health resources such as gloves, syringes, and needles. Fear of discrimination and the Filipino trait of fatalism result in lack of voluntary testing, inadequate reporting, and unquantifiable continuing sources of infection. As a consequence, the approach to the treatment of AIDS at the individual and societal level often is very inadequate.

References

Alora, A.T. (ed.). 1992. *Casebook in Bioethics*. Manila: Southeast Asian Center for Bioethics.
———. 1996. Ethics, AIDS and the healthcare provider. *Santo Tomas Journal of Medicine* (July/September), 87–91.
Ashley, B., and K. O'Rourke. 1989. *Healthcare Ethics: A Theological Analysis*. St. Louis: Catholic Health Association of the United States.
Boisaubin, E. V. 1991. Ethical and legal issues in the treatment of patients with AIDS. *Texas Medical Journal* (February), 76–80.
Council for Ethical and Judicial Affairs. 1988. Ethical issues involved in the growing AIDS epidemic. *Journal of the American Medical Association* 259 (March): 1360–61.

Dwyer, J. M. 1994. Managing HIV / AIDS with limited resources. *Proceedings of 4th WEST-PAC Congress of Infectious Diseases* (December), 100–101.

Mertz, D. M., A. Sushinsky, and Vao Schüklenk. 1996. Women and AIDS: The ethics of exaggerated harm. *Bioethics* 10: 93–113.

Ross, M. 1989. Psychological ethical aspects of AIDS. *Legal Medical Ethics* 15: 74–81.

Steinbrook, R., B. Lo, J. Tirpack, J. W. Dilley, and P. A. Volberding. 1985. Ethical dilemmas in caring for patients with AIDS. *Annals of Internal Medicine* 103: 787–90.

Zuger, A., and S. Miles. 1988. Physicians, AIDS and occupational risk. *Journal of the American Medical Association SouthEast Asia* (April): 47–51.

Human Organ Transplants

Danilo C. Tiong

Case

Pusakal, a 37-year-old Roman Catholic father of four, is an inmate in the maximum security section of the Philippine National Penitentiary. Convicted of premeditated murder, he has been in prison for the past two years, awaiting execution. His family has moved from their hometown in eastern Visayas to an area for slum-dwellers in metropolitan Manila. Their move was prompted in part by threats and intimidation directed against them by the family of his victim and in part by their wish to be closer to Pusakal.

Pusakal's wife, Dolor, is a laundrywoman; she also is sickly. Their only son died after being hit by a vehicle while selling cigarettes in the streets. No one else in the family is earning an income.

Pusakal has decided to sell his kidney to Trish Kram Park, a Korean national, for $3,000 to provide capital for his family to establish a small business and live on the profits. Included in the agreement of sale were the following conditions. First, Park's family would shoulder all of the hospital bills incurred. Second, they would pay for any medical expenses that would be incurred until Pusakal recovered from surgery. Third, in case of death or complications arising from the operation, Pusakal's family is to be compensated with an additional $1,000. Fourth, all of these conditions are to be carried out regardless of whether the transplant is successful.

This case is not an isolated one. Such circumstances are repeated often in the Philippine National Penitentiary. Inmates consider organ sales to be the best available option to remedy the financial distress of their families; they justify it as an act of bodily offering and sacrifice for the sake of family.

Elements of the Problem in the Religious and Moral Context

The Roman Catholic Church has taught that body parts are meant to function for, and are thus subordinated to, the good of the whole body. This principle of totality, however, allows for the removal of a part for the good of the whole, should that become necessary. The "whole" can be understood in the narrow sense of the person's physical body or the wider sense of the social corpus. Aside from this objective consideration, current Catholic moral theology allows organ donation out of love, provided that the functional integrity of the body is maintained. The action is justified by virtue of the charitable motives of the donor. Based on Christ's teaching (John 15:13), charity may even include heroic acts such as organ donation. Because such acts are heroic, they are not considered morally obligatory; they are licit as free and voluntary acts of charity.

The moral licitness of organ donation must link the motive of charity with the Church's norms concerning justice: Although one is obliged to give what is owed to another, one is not obliged to act beyond what is morally or physically very difficult. There are certain conditions for morally allowable organ donation. First, adequate safeguards must be taken so that the donor does not suffer serious harm. Second, as a consequence of the first, adequate safeguards should be taken so that the donor is not deprived of the functional integrity of his or her body. Third, the graver the nature of the sacrifice, the graver the reason must be for which the transplant is performed.

Organ sale, as opposed to donation, often appears to be morally objectionable because of the obvious risks of possible abuse, such as forced sale, as well as individual exploitation and degradation. Often there are alternative ways and means to earn an income aside from the sale of healthy organs.

Analysis

What can be said morally about Pusakal's organ sale? What values must be given close attention? Against the backdrop of Filipino culture, certain considerations seem to be morally relevant: family security and honor, parental responsibilities of provision and education as shared by husband and wife, and general conditions of economic employment (Harvey 1987).

Customarily, the Filipino husband assumes the role of provider. In this value-laden role, the Filipino male is expected to provide for his family, as best as he can, the basic requirements of food, shelter, clothing, and education. The Filipino wife traditionally has the sole role of manager of the home. Her primary responsibilities are doing household chores and rearing children. Mothers are solicitous and constantly protect their children. The mother teaches the children good manners and right conduct, including basic prayers and the importance of attending Sunday Mass.

Education also plays a strong role in the values of Filipino families. Every Filipino couple wants their children to obtain a college degree. Filipino parents will go to great lengths to be able to send their children to primary and secondary school as well and college, if possible. They take great pride in having children who are professionals. In fact, some parents consider the education of their children to be a form of inheritance. Education is a benefit that the family will attempt to provide.

Finally, it is considered a shame on the family for one of its members to acquire notoriety. One of the strong values of the Filipino family is to have a good moral reputation, particularly if the family is not influential or affluent.

Pusakal's peculiar circumstances invite comments regarding family, employment, and other values that are not altogether irrelevant or morally indifferent. Inside the National Penitentiary, opportunities available for inmates to generate income to support their families are severely limited, and the government does not provide for family support of prisoners. Although Pusakal may not want to, sooner or later he must join a gang, which will then function as his second "family." The mere act of accepting money from an inmate financier will identify Pusakal with that person's gang. Bound by *utang na loob* (gratitude) and *pakikisama* (cooperation), Pusakal must now become an active participant in all their intrigues and violence, conflicts and wars—many of them life-threatening. There is no middle ground of loyalties among prison inmates.

The Cultural Ethics at Work

Based on the simple facts of the case, as a human problem, the average Filipino cannot help but pose the problem in familial terms (Rosales 1987). As the family head, Pusakal has moral obligations to provide for family members. The fact that he is in prison does not absolve him of this responsibility. The fact that his wife cannot substitute for his role because of her illness and meager income only aggravates the situation and deepens his responsibility: Dolor's problems are not her problems alone; they are Pusakal's responsibilities as well.

For Pusakal, then, family is the key to understanding the problem; it also is the criterion of his ethical reasoning. The possibility of organ sale assumes its moral significance in this context. In Pusakal's mind, the organ sale will resolve most of his familial responsibilities. Given the circumstances, the extreme need of his family appears to outweigh the loss of one kidney. In fact, one could imagine Pusakal giving much more, if the situation demanded it. Subjectively, he senses a greater duty to his family's welfare than to his own well-being. His concern and love lighten the sacrifice he is making. There also may be a sense of resignation or fatalism in accepting the implications of living as an inmate. There is love and *utang na loob:* Pusakal recognizes the double burden on Dolor, who must be homemaker as well as provider, thereby assuming the social roles of both father and mother. Pusakal must protect Dolor, who would have difficulties finding other employment and could get even sicker or die, leaving the children in an even worse situation.

The kidney sale resolves Pusakal's obligations as provider in an extraordinarily fortuitous way. Unlike his previous efforts, this one-time provision of funds provides an excellent opportunity for them to survive decently—provided, of course, that they invest the money well and sustain the small business. They now have the means to live and even to obtain an education. Such provisions for the future are hardly trivial. Most important, Pusakal relives not only his family's misery but also its shame. The organ sale is an act of self-sacrifice, helping to redeem Pusakal of whatever moral turpitude he might have been guilty of by his crime.

Pusakal may not be aware that the Church typically considers selling a kidney to be morally unjustified and sinful (Ashley and O'Rourke 1986; O'Rourke and Brodeur 1986; Peschke 1978; Haring 1981; O'Donnell 1976). In Pusakal's mind, God—who sent His Son to save humans by sacrificing Himself—can only view Pusakal's own sacrifice in a benevolent light. Moreover, Pusakal did vow in marriage to show this kind of selfless love, a pledge of dedication to the family's welfare.

Of course, one might object that the end does not always justify the means. Granting that Pusakal's objective and motive are appropriate, the means may be morally illicit. Given his concrete circumstances, however, any alternatives are purely formal and theoretical; they are not realistic. Not only does his family's general economic situation provide limited alternatives, his status as an inmate reduces even those that could be imagined. The kidney sale may be considered an act of self-defense against the unjust aggression of poverty. Pusakal's choice takes advantage of the most efficient and effective means at his disposal, powered with the noble and morally acceptable motive of love. Absent the kidney sale, there is little likelihood that he could ever achieve such opportunities for his family.

Casting the problem in the framework of family demonstrates how trivial it would have been to reduce the moral concerns to merely monetary terms. Although the financial incentives appear to be decisive, the fundamental reasons for the sale are those on which cultural values insist. Money itself is not the objective; it is the instrumental means to the end. Material resources are only the means to obtain the real end: to liberate Pusakal's family from its economic misery. This case is structurally similar to a case in which Pusakal donates his kidney to another person, who then agrees to provide for Pusakal's family. The only difference in this case is that the purchase is outright, explicit, and honest.

Although many moral theologians consider Pusakal's choice an objectively grave mortal sin, his motives of love and charity, which are implicit in the organ sale, protect his moral integrity because the action is done for the most unselfish reasons. Pusakal's decision signifies honor, integrity, dignity, and life for his family and thus appears proportionate to the nature of the sacrifice. Perhaps, then, this case is better analyzed not under the norm of justice (Beauchamp and Childress 1989) but through the virtues of love and charity.

References

Ashley, B. M., and K. D. O'Rourke. 1986. Ethics of health care. *Catholic Health Association*, 155–59.

Beauchamp, T., and J. Childress. 1989. *Principles of Biomedical Ethics*, 3rd ed. New York: Oxford University Press.

Haring, B. 1981. *Free and Faithful*, vol. 3. New York: Seabury Press.

Harvey, J. C. 1987. Medical ethics: A summary analysis and application. *UNITAS* 60 (June), University of Santo Tomas, Manila.

O'Donnell, T. J. 1976. *Medicine and Christian Morality*. New York: Alba House.

O'Rourke, K. D., and D. Brodeur. 1986. *Medical Ethics: Common Ground for Understanding*. St. Louis: Catholic Health Association.

Peschke, C. H. 1978. *Christian Ethics*, vol. 2. Alcester and Dublin: C. Goodliffe Neale.

Rosales, V. J. A. 1987. Bioethical problems in the developing world. *UNITAS* 60 (June), University of Santo Tomas, Manila.

Death and Dying

Josephine M. Lumitao

Death is a fact of life that transcends cultural and racial boundaries. The mystery and finality of death can be understood by all people regardless of their creed, country of origin, or political affiliation. Despite death's universality, certain aspects of death are defined by the cultural, religious, economic, and medical environment. The central role of the family, the high costs of health care, the cultural traits of fatalism, *utang na loob* (debt of gratitude), caring, and the deep religiosity of the Filipino patient result in an interplay of factors that create situations that may conflict with Western ethical principles of autonomy and informed consent. This discussion of death in the developing world attempts to show that although the Filipino experience of facing death is superficially similar to the western European and North American ethos of dying, the Filipino experience is experientially fundamentally different.

The Dilemma of the Dying Patient

Current medical practice has been influenced by extensive technological progress. High-technology advancements have created a wide spectrum of treatment options, forcing health professionals to be very discriminating and prudent in employing such options for individual patients. Physicians must be acutely aware that although they can help the whole person in most cases, there will be some patients for whom they can aim only to provide psychological benefits, such as the maintenance of respiration, temperature, and blood pressure. The latter group of patients constitute a special category, carrying a unique set of bioethical concerns: They represent the dilemma of the dying patient.

Dying patients suffer from irreversible and extensive organic damage; medical science can offer no benefit to them. This general definition applies to a vast array of examples, such as the terminal cancer patient, the premature infant with multisystem underdevelopment and failure, or the patient with multiple organ failure resulting from progressive disease or acute causes. The bioethical challenges to which such cases give rise include determining when a patient is terminally ill; whether physicians should be fully truthful with dying patients or their families about the nature and extent of the patient's condition; and whether to withdraw extraordinary forms of medical treatment, as well as providing pastoral counseling and family support and the morality of euthanasia and physician-assisted suicide.

Understanding Life and Death

A person's concept of death is influenced by his or her concept of life. Largely shaped by religious tradition, Filipino Catholics regard life as a gift from God that is to be treasured and cherished. It has a value that is to be used for the service of God and others. For Filipino patients, this "other" refers in an immediate manner to members of one's family, one's group (*barkada*). Life does not represent an absolute value to be idolized, however. Consequently, when the time comes to relinquish or surrender life, Filipinos do so with a focus on the most important value: eternal life with God. Most Filipinos are deeply religious and have faith that God will somehow lighten the burden of facing death.

When maintaining life imposes extreme physical, psychological, or financial burdens on a patient or the patient's family, determining whether death is imminent and if current health care treatments are extraordinary and therefore nonobligatory is vital. Given the authority of the Filipino physician, a great deal of emphasis is placed on the ethical beliefs of the physician. Filipino patients look to their physicians for medical as well as moral advice. At times, this attitude leads to inappropriate consequences. For example, some physicians advise patients and their families to prolong life at all costs. This observation is common in the Philippines, where many practitioners believe that life belongs to God alone and that only He can take it away. This attitude typically results in overly aggressive treatment of the patient and significant financial burden to the family.

Truth-Telling

One of the main issues in the care of a dying patient is whether the patient should be told the truth about his or her terminal condition. Most western European and North American theories of bioethics argue that competent patients must be told the truth so that they can exercise autonomous decision making to put their affairs in order as their biological life ends. Alternatively, some theorists argue that the moral permissibility of truth-telling depends on the balance of benefits versus harms, where fully informing patients of their condition is thought to provide more benefits than costs.

Such practices are significantly different in the Philippines. The close family ethos that reaches out to care for the needs of a sick patient, especially a dying one, protects the family member from the stress of knowing his or her diagnosis or having to make stressful decisions while preparing to die. During such times, the dominant family figure or several family members approach the physician and ask about the diagnosis, then decide on treatment options. Usually, they even specifically request that the physician shield the patient from the harmful effects of knowing the truth. The family simply takes over. This general disregard for Western ideals of autonomy and the consequent loss of confidentiality is totally alien to most contemporary accounts of Western bioethics. Yet it is the standard of care in the Philippines. Occasionally, patients will ask about their illness. Here, the Filipino trait of seeking peace and harmony at all costs and the cultural aspects of caring become evident. The harsh truth will be stated as pleasantly as possible—and always with an optimistic note of trust in God's providential care.

For example, cancer patients will never be told directly that there is a malignancy. The situation will be communicated in euphemisms such as "you have a *bukol* (mass) that requires an operation—but do not worry, we will do our best to take care of you." Such statements may not be entirely adequate, under Western standards, for the patient to make an informed decision, but they generally are considered adequate and morally appropriate from the Filipino point of view. After all, the patient usually does not make medical decisions; the family does. Moreover, fully honest and frank statements would be considered impolite and morally inappropriate.

Once the family and the physician agree on treatment options, patients rarely understand that they are dying until they grow progressively weaker. Even then, the average Filipino patient will not ask for the real diagnosis or hold a grudge against the physician for failing to tell the truth. The lack of information is interpreted as concern for the patient's well-being. Patients read between the lines, accepting the situation with mixed feelings of religious trust and a fatalistic resignation to events that are beyond their control. Typically, patients eventually learn their diagnosis—but in a manner that is culturally acceptable.

The strong religiosity of Filipinos is very evident with dying patients; at death, they often are surrounded by all sorts of religious images and objects. Families request more frequent visits, as well as confession and communion with chaplains. Some invite faith-healers to come to the hospital (with the physician's permission). Close relatives and members of the extended family take turns visiting the patient, but as the end draws near the patient and/or the family asks for anointing (i.e., extreme unction or sacrament of the sick) and permission to take the patient home. Dying patients generally want to die at home, surrounded by loved ones in familiar surroundings rather than in the impersonal, technological efficiency of hospitals. Significant secularization has somewhat altered this attitude; family members in urban areas occasionally prefer to have the patient remain in the hospital.

Withdrawal of Treatment

The Roman Catholic Church's teachings on withdrawal of treatment guide such decisions in dying patients. Extraordinary/disproportionate forms of treatment are therapies that, in the patient's or family's judgment, do not offer reasonable hope of benefit or entail excessive burdens (psychological, physical, or financial) on the patient or the family. In the Philippines, the high cost of health care must be borne almost exclusively by the family. After any significant expenses, such high costs qualify most treatment for dying patients as extraordinary. Justification for withdrawal of treatment on financial grounds is not difficult.

At times, however, the cultural traits of fatalism—interpreted as a desperate religious trust and a shrinking away from responsibility—cause a family to request that everything possible be done, without thought to the economic burden. Some just pray for a miracle and hope that the financial problem will resolve itself. Occasionally, however, the authoritarian health care provider is the one who insists that everything should be done in spite of the burdens this course of treatment will impose on the family. Such situations contribute to the financial problems that health care institutions bear and to the poor allocation of scarce resources. Education in ethical decision making and prudent judgment can minimize such difficulties.

Euthanasia

Euthanasia is an action or omission that in itself and by intention causes the death of the patient, usually to relieve suffering. Religious beliefs about the meaning of suffering (particularly its expiatory and redemptive value) and acceptance of one's fate make euthanasia an unacceptable option in Filipino health care. Patients' families typically are concerned about the moral permissibility of withdrawing extraordinary forms of treatment. The caring atmosphere of the family and the compassionate health care provider, strengthened by spiritual support from the chaplain, provide little room for thoughts of euthanasia. The Christian belief that death is not the end but only the beginning of an eternal life with the Father provides strength to the dying.

Conclusion

Cultural values and customs shape the ways in which persons face the universal reality of death. In the Philippines, the primacy of the family's role in decision making supersedes western European and North American concerns about autonomy. Religious beliefs and the cultural trait of fatalism make acceptance of death easier. On one hand, withdrawal of extraordinary forms of treatment may be easier because of the financial burden such treatment imposes on the patient's family. On the other hand, such fatalism sometimes results in an insistence on the provision of useless treatment. Rigid, unguided religious beliefs of an authoritarian health care provider may compound such difficulties. Moreover, although Filipino health care providers aim to provide compassionate care for the dying patient even when a cure is no longer possible, they must remember that they also bear the burden of supporting the family during this difficult process.

CASE 1: Mrs. A., a 68-year-old, active, independent, and cheerful grandmother who smokes heavily, is admitted to the hospital because of difficulty in breathing. Diagnostic tests reveal widespread, inoperable metastatic carcinoma of the lungs. Mrs. A. is expected to live only a few more months. Her devoted husband, children, and the chaplain are informed of the diagnosis. The family insists that Mrs. A. not be told the diagnosis, so that her remaining time at home will be as happy as possible. The physician and the nurses accept this decision. Mrs. A., however, says, "I have the feeling that something is being kept from me. I believe that I have the right to know what is wrong with me."

ANALYSIS: This case offers a typical example of the family taking over the autonomy of the individual patient in the decision-making process. Mrs. A. is an unusual patient from the Filipino perspective, however, because she asks for her diagnosis. Viewing this case from within Filipino culture, however, Mrs. A. as a grandmother is a figure of authority. The matriarchal focus in Filipino culture is significant. The divergence between the family's wishes and the wishes of a patient who happens to be an authority figure is very evident. The health care provider can ascertain whether Mrs. A. really wants to know by discussing directly with her her reasons for the request. Ascertaining that her request is that of a competent patient, the health care provider should convince the family of the benefits of informing Mrs. A. For example, the physician should explain that the information could be provided in stages, with pauses to ascertain its impact on Mrs. A.'s psychological status. Moreover, informing the patient would allow Mrs. A. time to prepare spiritually for her death.

CASE 2: Mr. C., a 17-year-old male, is the victim of a vehicular accident on his way to attend midnight mass at Christmas. He has suffered complete cord transection, upper cervical level, and is totally paralyzed from the neck down, requiring a ventilator to breath. His family requests that they be allowed to take him home after two weeks because of the mounting hospital bills, but his physician refuses, arguing that the only reason Mr. C. is still alive after all this time is because of God's will. Therefore, the physician asserts, Mr. C. will likely recover. The hospital bills reach P700,000 after 30 days, and when the owner of the jeep that hit Mr. C. refuses to pay the bills, Mr. C. is transferred to the charity ward. Mr. C.'s mother is a laundrywoman; his father is a writer who earns P3000 a month, and he has six younger siblings. Previously, Mr. C. augmented the family income by selling newspapers.

Mr. C.'s mother takes care of him in the hospital, practically living on the ward. As a result, care of the other siblings suffers. Indeed, his mother often ambu-bags him manually. When the bioethics committee consulted by the new attending physician informs Mr. C.'s family that he would need a respirator for the rest of his life, Mr. C. looks sad. After a few days, he requests that the respirator be removed. In contrast, his mother is indecisive.

ANALYSIS: This case offers an example of a patient whose death is imminent without the implementation of costly and permanent medical technology. Such care can be understood as extraordinary and thus nonobligatory treatment because it imposes an excessive and unreasonable financial burden on the patient's family. Mr. C.'s participation in the decision-making process, even though he is a minor, can be understood because he is the eldest child. His decision should be understood as a sacrifice for the good of the family, which is being torn apart by the financial and psychological burdens of his sickness. His mother's inability to decide is fully understandable: She is torn between wanting to give whatever is humanly possible to her son and realizing the burden this situation imposes on the rest of the family. She should be reassured, however, that although the withdrawal of treatment is a painful decision, it is the best for Mr. C. and the family.

Unfortunately, the authoritarian physician imposed his own beliefs on the patient, distorting the pattern of decision making and resulting in unnecessary expenses for the patient's family—as well as for the health care institution.

PART V

Allocation and Justice

Allocation of Scarce Resouces:
Macro-, Meso-, and Micro-Level Concerns

Angeles Tan Alora and Josephine M. Lumitao

Current systems of health care allocation in the developed and developing worlds do not provide access to adequate care for all patients. Whenever needs exceed resources, health care must be prioritized. Such decisions take place at the macro, meso, and micro levels. Macro-allocation involves policy decisions about the distribution of resources on a social level, meso-allocation determines broad institutional decisions regarding resource usage, and micro-allocation sets local or individual unit usage. In each case, one must consider whether the available resources will be used to fulfill a limited set of basic needs for a large number of people or to address the extensive needs of only a few individuals (i.e., low-cost/high-yield versus high-cost/low-yield allocation strategies).

The maldistribution of health care—whether it involves personnel, facilities, or supplies—is magnified in the Philippines. Big cities have tertiary hospitals with all the modern equipment, the best-trained health care providers, and the latest therapeutic modalities. In 1996, metropolitan Manila had 169 tertiary hospitals in a perimeter of 63,000 hectares—a superfluity. Western Mindanao, by contrast, had 78 hospitals in a total land area of 1,599,734 hectares. Remote areas have none. Because of limited government services, some Filipinos never have an opportunity to visit a physician. There is one nurse per 16,061 persons and one health worker per 33,670 persons in rural areas (National Statistical Coordination Board 1997). Even in areas where hospitals and health care providers are present, they often are not accessible to the poor. Poor Filipinos cannot afford the price of medications, the price of transportation to the physician's office, and the lost earnings while they receive health care.

The issue often lies in the choice of fundamental values, goals, and attitudes—deontological or utilitarian—that influence and determine allocations of the national budget to health care and distribution of these funds to various sectors of society.

In the Philippines, the goal of the government has been to increase economic progress and development. Poverty and ignorance cause Filipinos to place a low value on health. Justice, fairness, and equality as understood by

Westerners are nebulous for the Filipino because of varying and contradict-ing political images and slogans. There is no clear opinion concerning what is desirable and no clear vision of what should be attempted. This situation might explain our problems with macro-allocation. Competing undercurrents cause affirmative action to fail or do poorly. Abstract Western views of justice and fair allocations often have little force.

Cultural commitments of *pakikisama, hiya, utang na loob,* and *lusot* are ap-plied by health care policymakers in guiding allocations at the macro and micro levels (Andres 1988). At times this cultural milieu has significant costs. Person-alism affects the choice of beneficiaries, and needs dictate practicality. Many Filipinos may die as the result of the allocation of resources to favored persons and projects, though some survive in spite of scant available health care. This situation may be considered unfair and unjust, or it may be regarded as the un-fortunate outcome of more than moderate scarcity and the limits of any moral approach to allocation.

CASE 1: Traditional Birth Attendants

Delia, a 36-year-old mother, comes to the hospital because of moderate vagi-nal bleeding. She delivered her fourth child one day earlier, assisted by the tra-ditional birth assistant (TBA, or *hilot*). When she continued to bleed, the TBA advised her to go to a hospital.

Upon learning of Delia's medical history, the medical intern becomes in-dignant. She reprimands Delia for delivering with a TBA instead of coming to the hospital. She says the situation could have been prevented.

ANALYSIS: This case demonstrates the tension between scientific and tra-ditional medicine and its impact on the use of limited resources. The intern sees herself as an authority because of her scientific training. She fails to rec-ognize the contribution of the TBA, who was in authority in this case and who provided inexpensive, accessible health care.

Many mothers deliver in hospitals where hospitals are accessible. Where the hospital is too far, too expensive, or otherwise too threatening, however, mothers give birth with a TBA. A TBA generally is efficient, provides home service, has a good bedside manner, and is less costly. She also serves as coun-selor, adviser, companion, and family friend. In addition, the home is the best place to welcome a new baby. It is affordable, and it encourages family mem-bers to be around to provide support.

The TBA as a health care provider is an essential member of the health care team that reaches out to people for whom other levels of health care are inac-cessible. She provides a service that cannot be provided where nurses and physi-cians are unavailable. Yet many physicians—especially obstetricians—resent the

TBAs and even lobby against bills that might formally integrate them into the health care service. Because of *pakikisama* and *utang na loob* to the obstetricians, politicians might vote against such bills, to the detriment of the many poor.

The TBA should be regarded as a partner and colleague in assisting birth deliveries. Her role should be appreciated, not undermined; recognized, not ignored; and valued, not derided.

CASE 2: Rural Service

Dr. T. agrees to join the rural service to help the people. In the first week of practice, he sees three patients with pulmonary tuberculosis and one with malaria. He has been trained to do sputum smears and thick blood smears, but no microscope is available in his rural service. There also is no ultrasound for potentially complicated pregnancy. After one month, Dr. T. decides to return to the city to practice there.

ANALYSIS: To reach underserved areas, the Department of Health has provided various incentives for physicians. The Department offers a good salary, opportunities to go to the city for continuing medical education, and other benefits. Neither the attractive incentive package nor an appeal to patriotism compensates, however, for the unsafe environment, poor standard of living, and lack of modern facilities.

Aid to underserved areas must be approached holistically. It is not simply a matter of offering an attractive package to physicians; it also entails providing them with adequate technology, support, and assurance of a safe environment. There are not enough resources to meet all these goals, however.

CASE 3: Managed Care

Managed care has been presented as a possible approach for better resource use. The Philippines was the first country in Asia to adopt managed care. Private-sector initiatives have spawned a rapidly growing health maintenance organization (HMO) industry that has replaced traditional indemnity insurance as the favorite among corporate benefits managers. There are now 32 private HMOs operating in the country. The markets being served and targeted by managed care organizations are mainly the employed sector and the growing middle class. There is no attempt to serve the lower economic class.

ANALYSIS: Low-cost health care plans can offer basic, affordable outpatient and inpatient benefits. Outreach to large segments of the low-income population has been started. If the plan is successful, it may considerably reduce the number of people who depend on government-funded services. This reduction in demand will free limited government resources to be diverted to the smaller indigent segment of the population. This transition requires Filipinos to accept a lower standard of health care, however, to make it affordable. It cannot guarantee the same access to technologies or expensive drugs.

CASE 4: Meso-Allocation within Religious Hospitals

While setting up a program on the state of Catholic hospitals that are run by priests and nuns, a television journalist discovers significant polarization within a hospital between the religious brothers and a sizable group of the staff. Some of the nursing staff complain that their training is less than complete with regard to specific procedures such as abortion, tubal ligation, sterilization, and so forth. This lack of training puts them at a disadvantage when they finish their training and transfer elsewhere. On the other hand, the brothers are adamant that certain procedures are incompatible with the religious nature of the hospital.

Part of the difficulty is that residents and consultants refer abortions and similar cases to themselves, at their second office on the other side of town (at the Protestant hospital). The brothers are aware of this practice and would prefer to terminate their services except that no replacement physicians are available. Moreover, the consultants and residents are uncomfortable with the fact that the sisters and brothers forgo their professional fees when treating indigent patients. This practice, they argue, causes them to lose face. The brothers and sisters counter that the physicians are heartless for refusing to behave likewise. An additional point of conflict is that the secular physicians and nurses find many excuses to avoid attending religious activities at the hospital—such as retreats, eucharistic celebrations, and other liturgical services, as well as lectures related to professional and medical ethics.

ANALYSIS: Religious hospitals have the moral authority to insist on preserving the religious character of their hospital. The predominantly Roman Catholic character of the Philippines means that certain services that Western medicine takes for granted, such as abortion and sterilization, will not be available in all health care institutions—nor will training for such procedures be provided. Such resource allocation is an appropriate institutional means of preserving the traditional religious values of the Filipino culture.

CASE 5: Micro-Allocation Based on Familial Relations

A physician friend of the chairman of the department of obstetrics and gynecology obtains a private donation of P500,000 with the stipulation that it should be used to purchase a fetal monitor. The physician friend has a son who is a staff member of the same department and who recently completed a fellowship in high-risk obstetrics. The other staff members argue that the department urgently needs its own blood bank. They argue that the money would be better used to set up the department's own blood bank; the remaining funds could be utilized to improve prenatal care, such as providing free iron tablets and nutrition lectures.

ANALYSIS: In the Philippines, the combined cultural traits of family kinship, personalism, and *utang na loob* (debt of gratitude) require certain allocation decisions to be made in favor of one's family or a person to whom a debt is owed. Moreover, allocation decisions that are based on the health care needs of patients also should be balanced with the commitment and obligation of health care institutions to educate and train skilled physicians, nurses, and technicians. Such training sometimes will require access to expensive technology to keep the staff abreast of significant developments.

The conflict in this case illustrates the tension between different kinds of needs. The argument for utilizing the donation to establish a blood bank and improve prenatal care is that this approach represents a low-cost/high-yield scheme that will serve more patients. Maternal mortality in the Philippines is related to the following factors: hemorrhage, 32 percent; hypertensive disorders of pregnancy, 31 percent; infection, 27 percent; and other factors, 10 percent. Each of these causes often is preventable, if detected early, with inexpensive prenatal screening mechanisms. On the other hand, deciding to purchase a fetal monitor is an example of a high-cost/low-yield allocation scheme that caters to the needs of a limited group of patients. Yet the monitor also fulfills the obligations of the institution to the continuing education and training of its health care staff.

The stipulation that the donation be used to purchase a fetal monitor—with the "incidental" fact that the person who obtained the funds has a son who would benefit from this choice—may appear unacceptable from an impersonal Western moral perspective. It is perfectly acceptable, however, from the Filipino point of view. Within the Filipino context of family kinship, caring and personalism, a sense of duty, and responsibility and loyalty to persons from one's own family, the action is even praiseworthy. Again, one finds the moral focus on obligations to persons rather than commitments to abstract, impersonal principles (Gorospe 1988).

References

Andres, T. D. 1988. *Understanding Filipino Values*. Manila: New Day Publishing.

Gorospe, V. 1988. *Filipino Values Revisited*. Quezon City: National Bookstore, Inc.

National Statistical Coordination Board. 1997. *Philippine Statistical Yearbook*. Makati City, The Philippines: National Statistical Coordination Board.

Ethical Issues in Research

Angeles Tan Alora

Efficient and effective research presents unique challenges in the developing world. Poverty and ignorance are the main factors that limit research in the Philippines. Although the Philippine Council for Health Research Development provides funding, most of the available funds are awarded to government institutions. Research methodology is not emphasized in undergraduate medical education, nor is research a priority in the academic field. Because private researchers fear stringent requirements for submitting a research proposal or are unable—through ignorance or lack of institutional support—to write an acceptable research proposal, they often fail to submit or receive approval of research proposals, thereby depriving themselves of financial support. The limited availability of funds also circumscribes the number of subjects, as well as available screening and monitoring procedures.

Although some institutions carefully evaluate research protocols with bioethics committees and institutional review boards to approve research proposals, most do not. Research in private institutions often is subsidized by drug companies and usually consists of clinical trials. The Philippines is a popular site for clinical drug trials. Compared to developed countries, willing subjects for such trials are plentiful, requirements are less stringent, expenses are low, and government monitoring is minimal. Alternatively, cheaper descriptive studies are carried out, rather than expensive experimental studies. That is, rather than developing an experimental protocol, researchers will report clinical outcomes and publish case vignettes. In either case, the topics frequently are not very relevant for national health care needs.

The concern is that research subjects are being exploited. Subjects typically come from the charity wards of hospitals, employees of institutions where research is undertaken, or other disadvantaged groups. Researcher subjects are not adequately informed about potential risks to ensure free and informed consent. Although subjects give permission to be involved in research, the amount of information conveyed about the research may be restricted. Moreover, whereas such research may produce significant profits for the pharmaceutical companies, subjects do not receive an equitable share of the benefits of the research.

In terms of Filipino culture, *pakikisama* affects the way research protocols are written. It also significantly affects the form of publication. If conclusions are harmful to certain stakeholders, they are not made public, or they are phrased in very mild or neutral terms. Poorly conducted research often is published, simply because editors feel that they are unable to refuse to publish submitted papers.

One result is that careful, scientifically rigorous research is rare. Only a minority of researchers take pride in what they do and do it well. These researchers usually have benefited by having sufficient research funds and the professional expertise to conduct research.

CASE 1: The Attending Physician/Researcher

Marina is admitted to a charity ward because of community-acquired pneumonia. Sputum examination reveals streptococcus pneumonia that is sensitive to a variety of antimicrobials. Penicillin is the drug of choice, but Marina has no money to buy it.

The resident informs Marina that she will be given a new drug that is not yet available on the market; the drug will be free because the organism is likely sensitive to it. Marina is grateful; she takes the new drug—a broad-spectrum antibiotic on clinical trial—and gets well. The resident has another case to add to his study.

ANALYSIS: Some people worry about abuse or exploitation of the poor. For Marina, receiving no medicine may mean death, whereas obtaining a 4th-generation cephalosporin means life, even with some risk and adverse effects. Weighing the benefit/risk ratio favors taking the drug. Including Marina as a research subject is not exploitative; it is aiding Marina.

In the Filipino culture, physicians often make such decisions. As in this case, the researcher—who presumably also is Marina's attending physician—decided that receiving the drug is in her best interests, even though she will not be fully informed of its risks. His paternalistic attitude is a *lusot* from obtaining free and informed consent. If Marina is not informed of the risks, she cannot give informed consent. She is vulnerable because of her impoverished state and dependent relationship. In addition, cultural considerations of *hiya* place significant pressure on the patient not to withhold consent. True concern for Marina's interests should not be limited to providing her with the drug because it may help her; such concern should extend to the physician's behavior in interacting with Marina. Specifically, the physician/researcher should show respect for Marina as a person—which requires explaining to her the positive and negative aspects of taking the drug and asking if she understands the consequences of her choice.

Although Marina benefits from receiving the free drugs, she also should benefit from contributing to the success of the research. Without subjects, there could be no research. Large budgets provide funds for medications, laboratory procedures, and research staff. The budget also should include an equitable share of income for the research subjects. Too often, poor or marginalized subjects are "forced" to subsidize rich and powerful researchers. The subjects agree to take the risks and settle for less than they deserve because they do not know any better. This situation reflects poorly on those in authority.

Eagerness to be part of a multi-center and often international trial may make the researcher overlook testing defects, such as nonrandom selection of subjects and limited screening and monitoring procedures, which may support false conclusions. Researcher and institutional integrity is at stake.

CASE 2: The Professor as Researcher

A medical school professor is doing a study on a hepatitis B vaccine. After lecturing her class about hepatitis B, she announces the subject of her research. Students who volunteer pay a discounted rate for the vaccine and have free antibody titers performed before and after vaccination. The professor enrolls all volunteers in her office.

ANALYSIS: This situation is an example of an authority figure requiring obedience. *Hiya, pakikisama*, respect for authority, and the dependent relationship of students make refusing to volunteer very difficult for the students.

This recruitment process was the easiest way to obtain volunteers. Many were immediately available at no economic cost. Justifying such recruitment policies by saying that volunteers benefited because of the discounted rate is another form of *lusot*.

CASE 3: Employee / Research Subject

Clara, a clerk in the university, hears from friends that the pharmacology department is paying volunteers for a research study. Clara goes to the department, where a research aide explains to her that a physician (whose name Clara knows and respects) is trying to determine how much of a particular drug is left in the blood after 24 hours. For the study, 10 cc of blood is extracted, two tablets of this "safe" drug are swallowed, and the following day another 10 cc of blood is extracted. Clara will receive P150 (equivalent to her daily wage) after the second blood sample is drawn. Clara is satisfied with the explanation and happy about the arrangement, and she volunteers for the experiment.

ANALYSIS: The researcher, through the research aide, has failed to communicate adequately and made *lusot*. When Clara neglects to ask for information, the aide withholds it. In addition, the money offered may unduly influence Clara.

Money can be used as a motivating factor. In a country in which poverty is rampant and many people need money, financial rewards may be used as an incentive to acquire subjects for a study, provided risks are minimal. Even if risks are more than minimal, one can easily cite conditions in which the benefits money can bring can make becoming a research subject cost-effective. As long as benefits and risks are clearly understood, the choice should be left to the subject, although we must recognize that at times there is really no choice.

A Tax on Luxury Health Care, Generic Drugs, and a Proposal for a New Preferential Option for the Poor

Angeles Tan Alora

For the individual Filipino, health is not a priority. Financial resources are spent on food, shelter, clothing, education, and even entertainment rather than health care. Health becomes an important consideration only when it is lost. In general, medical care is understood as curative rather than preventive (Gorospe 1988). The same psychology prevails among lawmakers. Approximately 28 percent of the national budget (P11,470 billion) is allocated for health. This figure represents P167 ($6) per person—0.003 percent of the per capita health budget in Germany and 0.002 percent of per capita health spending in the United States.

Because the national budget is unable to provide sufficient funds for health care, alternative schemes to supplement these limited resources should be developed. One possibility would be to impose additional fees on those who seek and can afford to purchase luxury care (such as private hospital rooms, elective surgery, physician choice, and nongeneric medications) to provide funds for health care for those who have none. A tax on luxury health care probably would raise significant financial support for impecunious care. Moreover, such a tax need not be limited to governmental initiatives or the Philippines. Institutions throughout the developing world could cost shift in this manner to extend their ability to care for the poor.

CASE 1: Rich Subsidizing Poor

St. Tomas Hospital has two divisions: private and clinical. Upper-class patients are admitted into the private division, which has individual, air-conditioned rooms; poor patients are admitted to the clinical division wards—which have significantly less privacy and electric fans. Costs for procedures, medicines, and professional care are considerably higher in the private division than in the clinical division. Profits from the private division are partially used to subsidize the clinical division.

ANALYSIS: This arrangement is an example of resource sharing. Rich patients must pay the price for the special services and attention they desire. Those who can afford to purchase care in the private health sector are obliged to support (through the higher fees they are charged) those who are only able to afford government or charitable sectors. Some observers may cry "unfair." In the Filipino culture, however, *pakikisama* and *utang na loob* will prevent rich patients from complaining. Out of *pakikisama* and generosity, they will be more than willing to share. Out of *utang na loob* to the health care giver, they will not complain.

CASE 2: The Generics Law

The generics law was passed to make medicine affordable for the poor. It ordered that all prescriptions be written using generic names, that pharmacies offer to consumers a listing of generic drugs and their prices, and that consumers choose which product to buy. Many physicians opposed the generics law. They felt that it meant losing their professional right to prescribe their choice of medication.

ANALYSIS: Many physicians and patients choose expensive imported brands. This pattern is partially related to deeply ingrained cultural beliefs. The Philippines was under Spanish rule for 400 years, and then significant American influence for another 100 years. This history has resulted in a "colonial mentality," a mindset that regards imported and expensive products as better, whereas products that are made locally and inexpensively are considered inferior. Hence, when physicians prescribe drugs, many prefer imported brands; and when patients purchase drugs, they do not necessarily choose the cheapest product.

Even if patients are convinced by the Department of Health education campaign of the bioequivalence of generic drugs, many are not ready to usurp the physician's authority to choose. The cultural undercurrents of respect for authority and *pakikisama* prevent the generics law from succeeding on a practical level. An alternative might be to allow anyone who wants to use non-generic drugs to do so, but to impose an additional tax on them. This tax could be used to subsidize generics for the poor.

In general, health care expenditures in the Philippines indicate that too much money is being spent on medications and drugs. In 1986, the Department of Health expressed concern about the country's health care expenditure pattern. The relationship between physicians and the pharmaceutical industry in the Philippines has come under scrutiny because of the excessive use of drugs. According to a study by the Asian Development Bank in 1985, nearly 50 percent (US$355 million) of the total health expenditure for that year (US$762.9 million) was spent on pharmaceuticals. Yet an analysis of patterns of primary causes of morbidity and mortality, diarrhea, and respiratory infections suggests that the Philippines could achieve better health at a lower cost by making improvements in public sanitation. The experience of industrialized countries supports this claim. At the turn of the 20th century, before the advent of antibiotics, these countries achieved a marked decline in the incidence of infectious and communicable diseases by improving sanitation (Miranda 1992). In the Philippines, the emphasis remains on prescribing medications; the drug industry promotes this practice with marketing tactics aimed at physicians. There has been significant resistance to efforts to encourage the use of less-costly generic drugs. All parties—including health professionals, drug industry personnel, and consumers—need to be educated about the very real problem of excessive spending and learn about other possible solutions.

Do we spend as much as we do on drugs because they are very expensive or because we are using them excessively? The cost of drugs undeniably is spiraling. This trend has been attributed to the fact that 95 percent of the materials used in the production of drugs are imported; therefore, they are subject to fluctuating conditions in the foreign market. A 1976 study of the pharmaceutical industry in our region by the United Nations-Asian and Pacific Development Institute (UNAPDI) assessed drug utilization patterns on the basis of morbidity estimates and Western pharmaceutical therapy standards (UNAPDI 1976). The study found that consumption of antibiotics and analgesics in the Philippines is approximately 300 percent of the required amount; consumption of cough and cold preparations is 150 percent of the required amount. A recent survey of physicians in Southeast Asia, including the Philippines, revealed that only approximately 2 percent of physicians prescribe a single product to patients during a visit (*Drug Monitor* 1989). Apparently, drugs are utilized for conditions that do not necessarily warrant their use.

Given these circumstances, the government launched its National Drug Policy program, through which it hoped to make essential drugs available to a greater proportion of the population. Part of this program is the campaign for rational and pragmatic use of drugs. This objective is based on a report to the World Health Organization (WHO) that shows that a significant reduction in expenditure on drugs (up to 70 percent) can be achieved through rational drug therapy (WHO 1988). The Generics Act was passed in 1988 to fully implement the national drug policy. This law requires that prescriptions use the international nonproprietary name of the drug to allow patients to select from less-expensive (generic) preparations of the same drugs. Even before this law was passed, the Philippine Medical Association (PMA) expressed objections to certain provisions of the law. The PMA had the following concerns:

- Uncertainty about the ability of the Bureau of Food and Drug to ascertain the bioequivalence of new generic drugs before they are licensed for marketing
- Indiscriminate substitution of drugs prescribed for conditions such as heart failure, endocrine disorders, or fertility disorders might result in different preparations from the ones originally prescribed, and such preparations might not achieve the desired effects in patients

The PMA contended that doctors should not be penalized for failing to comply with the law because their disobedience is based on concern for their patients. In recognition of the validity of these concerns, the Department of Health has a listing of drugs that may not be substituted. However, proponents of the Generics Act have expressed the belief that the opposition of the PMA is based solely on the "alliance" it has formed with the drug industry (*Drug Monitor* 1988, 1990; Tan 1991b).

These exchanges have brought to the forefront the relationship between doctors and the drug industry. This relationship has been described as a "productive alliance" (American College of Physicians 1990), as well as one characterized by "mutual distrust" (Alkinson et al. 1984). Although the terms "productive alliance" and "mutual distrust" are very different, both are appropriate to describe the relationship between physicians and the drug industry. Physicians and the drug industry are both part of the "humane" business of health care, but the nature of their involvement, their concerns, and their goals differ. The drug industry is motivated to make a profit, whereas the medical profession focuses on serving the interests of the patient.

The drug industry has come under a great deal of criticism because it serves a vulnerable population: Its consumers are ill. Remembering that the industry is motivated and driven by profit eliminates many of the false expectations we may have of pharmaceutical firms. WHO has developed guidelines on the ethical treatment of patients. The very structure of the pharmaceutical workforce, however, serves the industry's aggressive marketing tactics. Whereas other industries have only 11 percent of the workforce in nonproduction jobs, nearly 40 percent of the drug industry's personnel are nonproduction workers (mostly sales representatives) (*Ibon Primer Series* 1986). Drug sales promotion efforts focus on manipulating the prescribing habits of practicing physicians.

Despite discussion of an alliance between physicians and the drug industry generated by debates regarding the Generics Act, the PMA offered no statement regarding this specific accusation. Was this because there is no truth to the accusation or because there is something they have decided is better left unsaid? A series of articles about drugs criticized the medical profession for its ties with the pharmaceutical industry. Again, there was minimal response by physicians. In an attempt to correct the perception that physicians are apathetic toward this situation and these accusations, R. R. Angeles revealed that the PMA has long recognized the vulnerability of physicians to the drug industry and the possibility that this relationship may prevent physicians from always being objective and giving primary importance to their patients' best interests. Because of these questions, in 1973 the PMA promulgated "The Ethical Guidelines on the Relationship between the Drugs and Pharmaceutical Industry and the Practicing Physician" (Angeles 1983).

The medical profession's silence on this matter could be related to the Filipino aversion to direct confrontation. Several medical directors in the drug industry are members of academia. This arrangement has worked for the benefit of academia because it has provided support for many of its programs. In a situation such as ours in which there are very limited resources for non–income-generating activities, support from the drug industry has become invaluable. The relationship between physicians and the drug industry in the Philippines seems to have achieved a comfortable middle ground. This is not to say that the hard-sell tactics of the industry have not affected the prescribing habits of physicians. The aforementioned studies indicate that drug industry tactics have influenced the practice of medicine in our country. Consequently, there is a need for an education campaign to institutionalize rational drug therapy as part of the National Drug Policy.

The government's effort to reeducate our medical practitioners demonstrates the extent to which we have let our objectivity be influenced by the drug industry. How long have we been remiss—and at what cost to our patients? Since the Generics Act's implementation, critics have pointed out its failure to reduce the cost of drugs (1990 drug sales: US$546 million) (Tan 1991a). What these critics have overlooked is that generic drugs provide a cheaper alternative to more expensive brand names. The success of the Generics Act will depend on the support of consumers and physicians (Kralewski, Pitt, and Dowd 1983). Its continued failure to live up to the expectations of its proponents demonstrates that legislation alone cannot solve the problem. Not only must medical professionals encourage the use of generic drugs, consumers themselves must be educated so that they exercise their prerogative to choose the less-expensive generic drugs. Moreover, the experience of industrialized nations that improved the health of their populations by improving public sanitation before antibiotics were available suggests that drugs need not be the only or even the primary focus of health care in the Philippines.

CASE 3: The UST Kidney Transplant Unit

In 1969, the Santo Tomas University Hospital formed the UST Kidney Transplantation Unit. In the same year, the first renal transplant was performed under the direction of Dr. Domingo Antonio, Jr.; the second was performed the following year. In September 1970, in an article in the *Journal of the Philippine Medical Association*, Dr. Antonio wrote:

> In our country, kidney transplantation is always an expensive procedure. . . .
> The transplant patient will spend the rest of his/her life taking immunosuppressive drugs. . . . Transplant patients have to accept this high price for the prolongation of life.
>
> In a developing country like ours, it becomes a debatable issue whether this considerable amount of money would be better invested to maintain or improve the life of many needy persons, rather than to prolong for an undetermined number of years the life of a single chronic renal case. . . (Antonio 1970).

After three years and two more equally successful kidney transplants, the hospital administration discontinued the program. They did not consider such research and service justifiable in the midst of more urgent basic primary health care needs in the country.

ANALYSIS: Where should funds to finance organ transplants come from? How does one compare saving a single chronically ill patient with meeting the basic primary health care needs of many patients? Is the attitude whereby expensive procedures are left to countries that can afford them while countries that cannot afford them limit their programs to meeting their basic primary health care needs morally permissible?

Provision of basic health care needs helps many people; a kidney transplant unit helps only a few. From a utilitarian perspective, the former maximizes the good. Yet all persons have a right to health care. Choosing to provide primary health care over a kidney transplant unit appears to prioritize utility over rights. Providing basic health care needs caters to statistical persons. Transplanting a kidney caters to an identified patient who will be seen as well and grateful. Choosing the former prioritizes statistical over identifiable lives. Yet those statistical lives represent real people who will receive health care if resources are preserved carefully.

The Santo Tomas University Hospital, in line with its mission, chose to present an image of a socially conscious institute with preference for the poor rather than an advanced medical center providing the latest and best technology can offer. The hospital's decision to discontinue kidney transplants is commendable.

A paradox could occur in the apparent decision, however, if the funds that would have gone to primary care did not. Thus, the discontinuation of the Kidney Transplant Unit was not helpful and only led to death for patients who needed transplants. The result would be that a dedication to an image (i.e., as a socially conscious institution) leads to death for identifiable persons without discernible improvement of others—a policy that forsakes a patient's life to provide for the poor.

Even more unfortunate is that there was the option—which the hospital did not take—of adding a surcharge to kidney transplants that could be devoted to primary care. A forced tithe that was applied to health care for the poor would have been the better alternative. This procedure would have resulted in an effective praxis of solidarity, as well as additional resources for impecunious care.

References

Alkinson, A., et al. 1984. Universality and pharmaceutical industry cooperation: The need to plan for the future. *Clinical Pharmacology* 35: 431–37.

American College of Physicians. 1990. Physicians and the pharmaceutical industry. *Annals of Internal Medicine* 112: 624–26.

Angeles, R. R. 1983. The corruption of our doctors. *Times Journal* (May 17).

Antonio, D., Jr. 1970. Experience in kidney homotransplantation. *Journal of the Philippine Medical Association* 46, no. 9: 581–90.

Drug Monitor. 1988. PMA seeks international support. *Drug Monitor* 3, no. 10: 121–22.

———. 1989. Highlights of a survey of Southeast Asian physicians. *Drug Monitor* 4, no. 1: 29.

———. 1990. Position paper on proposed amendments to the Generics Act of 1988. *Drug Monitor* 5, no. 8: 92–99.

Gorospe, V. 1988. *Filipino Values Revisited.* Manila: National Book Store.

Ibon Primer Series. 1986. The Philippine drug industry. Manila: Ibon.

Kralewski, J. E., L. Pitt, and B. Dowd. 1983. The effect of competition on prescription-drug product substitution. *New England Journal of Medicine* 309: 213–16.

Miranda, D. M. 1992. *Buting Pinoy: Probe Essays on Value as Filipino.* Manila: Divine Word Publications.

Tan, M. L. 1991a. The pharmaceutical industry in 1990. *Drug Monitor* 6: 11–12.

———. 1991b. Health resources. *Health Alert* 7, no. 116–17: 49–63.

United Nations-Asian and Pacific Development Institute (UNAPDI). 1976. The pharmaceutical industry in Asian countries. UNAPDI Health Technical Paper no. 36, PHI 15. Bangkok: UNAPDI/UNIDO.

World Health Organization (WHO). 1988. Ethical criteria for medicinal drug promotion. Geneva: WHO.

The Virtues and Vices of Dumping

Angeles Tan Alora

In the context of international medical markets, "dumping" involves disposal—usually in a developing country—of surplus pharmaceuticals, medical devices, or even medical services. Goods or services that are abundant in one area are transferred to another area and sold at below-market price. At first glance, this practice offers many benefits. At the source, a surplus is corrected, the supply remains limited, and the market value is unchanged. In the area to which the product or service is transferred, a supply is available at lower than market value, so recipients benefit.

Yet dumping may be accompanied by undesirable consequences. An inferior dumped product might harm rather than benefit the recipient. At other times, the activity may have ulterior motives: to serve as a tax shelter, to provide a public image of generosity, to get rid of unwanted goods, to exploit an opportunity to obtain practice in the use of some medicinal, and generally to use recipients as means for the donor's ends. Health care equipment, supplies, and even services are "dumped" from the rich to the poor—from developed countries to developing countries.

CASE 1: Dumped Drugs

Surplus Drug Company, a giant multinational pharmaceutical firm, has developed a drug that has been remarkably successful in controlling hypertension. Unfortunately, some deaths were attributed to the drug, and the company was forced to withdraw it from the market. After incurring much more expense, Surplus Drug produced a safer version of the drug. The risk of death per year of treatment dropped from 1 in 100,000 to 1 in 500,000. The newer, safer drug is notably more expensive than the prototype.

To reduce its losses from the quantity of prototype drug on hand, Surplus Drug offers it to the Philippines free of charge—under certain conditions that are financially beneficial to the company (i.e., tax cuts). The potential market in the Philippines is the great number of poor people who could not afford the safer drug but otherwise would receive no treatment for their hypertension.

Without treatment, their likely mortality per year is orders of magnitude higher than with treatment.

ANALYSIS: *Dumping* is a pejorative description that implies that a pharmaceutical company—usually a multinational firm—is disposing of dangerous or less-safe drugs that are forbidden in developed countries by sending them to a poor developing country. Should the government of the developing country accept dumped drugs? Should it insist on equal practice for Filipinos vis-à-vis the citizens of the developed country, where the government prohibited the sale of the drug?

The company argues that the drug is a benefit to the developing country, inasmuch as the price of an alternative, safer drug is prohibitive for poor people. The risk is admitted, but the benefit justifies the risk. The choice is between making available a drug with a known risk factor or not having any useful drug for the great number of patients with a serious disease because only the rich minority can afford the newer, safer drug.

One might find a parallel in the higher safety requirements imposed on car manufacturers in the developed world, such as safety belts, air bags, and so forth. The same car will be sold in the developing world without these safety features, at a price that is acceptable to the potential buyer; the risk of danger to the impecunious customer will be greater, but it will be considered acceptable in the situation. Rich people have the option of buying the safer—and much more expensive—car.

Many options are available to the rich but not the poor in all areas of life: choosing a school for children, choosing a place to live, selecting recreation and entertainment. This situation is an accepted fact of life, as long as the discrepancies are not too great and the position of the poor is not too unacceptable.

In a country such as the Philippines, the alternative to an inferior, dumped drug is no drug at all for many of its poor; a dumped drug, even if inferior, should be welcomed as long as the risk is acknowledged because it provides an advantageous balancing of benefits and harms. The poor should accept the drug because, on balance, it offers benefit, rather than accept a policy in which the poor will be worse off. Prudence dictates the acceptance of such drugs. People are helped by a choice of the lesser evil in an unfortunate situation that is insoluble at the moment.

Policymakers may still consider to refuse dumped drugs. Their pride and emotions may induce them to view the action as humiliating and even insulting. After all, who do the citizens of the developed world think they are that they can throw their "crumbs" to the developing world? Why should the developing world be used as means to their ends?

A more honest evaluation would lead to the realization that using such drugs often leads to more benefit than harm for the population. The advantage to the giver (tax deduction, image enhancing, etc.) is not unfair because both sides benefit. A negative attitude toward "dumped" drugs might lead to loss of life. The question then arises of whether people who speak against dumped drugs are murderers: whether their pride stops the poor from getting needed drugs or their false rhetoric kills the poor just for middle-class satisfaction.

True, charity can humiliate the receiver, but in this imperfect world charity often benefits the receiver as well. The issue often is not the actual dumping, inasmuch as the dumping is beneficial. Provided that such "dumping" is accompanied by informed consent and recipients are treated with dignity, it might even be considered praiseworthy. The issue often is national or racial pride—a false pride that is akin to hypocrisy. In this case, the hypocrisy kills.

CASE 2: Dumping Students—The Medical Missions

Medical missions are organized by groups of doctors, nurses, and medical students. In cooperation with local organizations, these missions visit underserved areas to perform surgical procedures and provide medical care. Follow-up is provided by local practitioners. Students at a medical mission are given the opportunity to perform procedures they would not yet be allowed to perform in medical school. Patients receive less than the "standard" quality of care.

ANALYSIS: In the Philippines, where more than half of the population is below the poverty level and 60 percent never see a physician, such efforts to alleviate the suffering of the poor should be lauded. Usually, medical care is not an "all or nothing" matter—either the best or worthless. Even medical students who are providing less than the best care may be able to provide acceptable care. With proper supervision, they certainly can provide care that is better than no care.

A similar situation occurs when American surgical teams visit the Philippines, performing surgical procedures for free. They use the operating rooms of government hospitals, then leave postoperative care to local physicians. These visiting surgeons give of their time and expertise to help underprivileged persons who could never afford the fees of local hospitals and surgeons. Local practitioners may criticize such actions on the grounds that trainees are practicing on impecunious Filipinos or receiving free vacations. In some cases, such criticisms may be defensive reactions by embarrassed local doctors who are unable or unwilling to perform the same operations without charge. They should welcome the help offered by others and hang their heads in shame.

The brutal truth of the matter is that in the health care policy of the developing world, the choice often is between insisting on the standard of care established in the developed world—which will deny most of the poor any treatment—or accepting a double standard of health care: one for the middle class and rich and another for the poor. If one accepts the latter choice as inescapable, one must insist that while giving less than the best care, one still should remain committed to doing the best one can under less than optimal circumstances. Although the best can be the enemy of the good, while giving less than the best one should still commit the best of one's moral attention.

With respect to public policy, all governments should be working constantly to change social structures and bring about a more just social order in which no one will have to accept a lesser-evil solution (i.e., less than the standard level of care). At the same time, governments also must act responsibly and realistically with the resources they possess. This attitude is true global justice and social solidarity.

APPENDIX
Background Readings

In the Compassion of Jesus: A Pastoral Letter on AIDS

The Catholic Bishops' Conference of the Philippines

None of us lives for himself, and no one dies for oneself (Rom. 14:7-8)

If one part suffers, all the parts suffer with it. . . . You are Christ's body, and individually parts of it (1 Cor. 12: 26-27).

Our dear Sisters and Brothers in Christ:

These words of St. Paul strongly remind us that we are responsible for one another. They reverberate in the declaration of Vatican II: "The joy and hope, the grief and anguish of the peoples of our time, especially of those who are poor or afflicted in any way, are the joy and hope, the grief and anguish of the followers of Christ as well" (On the Church in the Modern World, no. 1). More recently the words are echoed by the Second Plenary Council of the Philippines in its clarion call for solidarity (PCP-II Acts and Decrees, e.g., no. 295).

Today the call for mutual caring and solidarity is more urgent than ever as we Filipinos face a threat of potentially more catastrophic proportions than volcanic eruptions, floods, and conflicts. The name of this threat—the Human Immunodeficiency Virus (HIV) and the Acquired Immune Deficiency Syndrome (AIDS)—or HIV-AIDS for short.

The AIDS Situation: A Pandemic

First identified in 1981, the dread disease has swiftly spread in the space of less than ten years to every continent of the world. It is truly a pandemic, ravaging millions of lives, the lives of those infected, of their families and other loved ones as well. It cuts across all geographical and cultural boundaries, all classes and ages, although the young generations are particularly hit.

While statistics from 1984 to October 1992 tell us that in the Philippines only 356 had been diagnosed as HIV infected, including 84 AIDS cases, health offi-

cials believe that the actual number is hidden behind fear of exposure and ostracism, stigma and shame.

AIDS is transmissible by exposure to HIV-infected blood through transfusions, administration of blood products, organ transplants from infected
donors, use of unsterilized, HIV-contaminated needles and other equipment
by drug users and in health care facilities. It can also be transmitted from an infected mother to her unborn child.

But the most common means of transmission is through promiscuous
sexual behavior.

To date, no known vaccine or cure is available to combat the disease. Those
who are infected with HIV will remain infected for life. Although they may live
for many years without symptoms, they will eventually develop serious illnesses
which will lead to death. The grim image of the Apocalypse comes almost in-
exorably to mind: "I looked, and there was a pale green horse. Its rider was
named Death" (Rev. 6:8).

Moral Reflection and Response

It is clear that the situation demands the pastoral care of the Church. For the
Church must continue the mission of Jesus. In announcing the Goods News of
salvation, in healing the sick, in forgiving sinners, in being compassionate with
the multitudes, Jesus showed what the Church must do. God's people must be
at the side of those who suffer. Especially for the needy and the suffering of
today, the Church must be the Compassion of Jesus.

Our ministry of compassion for the afflicted must overcome fears and prej-
udices. Jesus has shown us the way, through the manner in which He dealt with
lepers, the ostracized and "untouchables" of His time. "Moved with pity, He
stretched out His hand, touched the leper, and said to him, I do will it. Be made
clean" (Mk. 1:41).

For us, an encounter with people infected with HIV-AIDS should be a moment of grace—an opportunity for us to be Christ's compassionate presence
to them as well as to experience His presence in them.

1. Our first attitude must be to serve and minister. Those who contract HIV-
AIDS, whether by accident or by consequence of their own actions, carry with
them a heavy burden: social stigmatization, ostracism, and condemnation. Let
us reach out to them, welcome them, serve them, as Jesus did the sick of his
time. To attend to their pain is to attend to the whole Mystical Body, to attend
to Christ Himself Who is the Head.

If there has been any moral responsibility, we must be ready to say, as Jesus
to the sinner: "Neither do I condemn you. Go, from now on do not sin any-
more" (Jn. 8:11)

2. To help stem the spread of this dread disease, we as a Church must collaborate with other social agencies in providing factual education about HIV-AIDS. So extensive is the popular ignorance about the disease as to encourage an irresponsible cavalier and casual attitude to sexual relationships. And too many are the myths surrounding it as to prevent effective pastoral care for those afflicted.

3. Most of all, we need to recognize the moral dimension of the disease. Though medically the cause of the disease can be identified as a virus, our faith tells us that its cause and solution go beyond the physical.

We cannot ignore the possibility that through this pandemic the loving Lord may be calling us, his children, to profound renewal and conversion: "For whom the Lord loves, he disciplines; he scourges every son he acknowledges" (Heb. 12:6; cf. 1 Cor. 11:32; Prov. 3:11-12). HIV-AIDS and other calamities that visit us are not necessarily the punishment of a loving and forgiving God for our personal or collective sins. But we know that Nature itself has often its own unremitting laws of reward and retribution with regard to actions we take, freely or not.

4. The moral dimension of the problem of HIV-AIDS urges us to take a sharply negative view of the condom-distribution approach to the problem.

We believe that this approach is simplistic and evasive. It leads to a false sense of complacency on the part of the State, creating an impression that an adequate solution has been arrived at. On the contrary, it simply evades and neglects the heart of the solution, namely, the formation of authentic sexual values.

Moreover, it seeks to escape the consequences of immoral behavior without intending to change the questionable behavior itself. The "safe-sex" proposal would be tantamount to condoning promiscuity and sexual permissiveness and to fostering indifference to the moral demand as long as negative social and pathological consequences can be avoided.

Furthermore, given the trend of the government's family planning program we have a well-founded anxiety that the drive to promote the acceptability of condom use for the prevention of HIV-AIDS infection is part of the drive to promote the acceptability of condom use for contraception.

For the above reasons we strongly reprobate media advertisements that lure people with the idea of so-called safe-sex, through condom use. As in contraception, so also in preventing HIV-AIDS infection condom use is not a failsafe approach.

5. We cannot emphasize enough the necessity of holding on to our moral beliefs regarding love and human sexuality and faithfully putting them into practice. All these, in order to prevent the spread of the disease and to provide the foundations for effective and compassionate pastoral care for those afflicted.

Among these moral beliefs is the beauty, mystery and sacredness of God's gift of human love. It reflects the very love of God, faithful and life-giving. This marvelous gift is also a tremendous responsibility. For sexual love must be faithful, not promiscuous, it must be committed, open to life, life-long and not casual. This is why the full sexual expression of human love is reserved to husband and wife within marriage.

Monogamous fidelity and chastity within marriage—these are ethical demands, flowing from human love as gift and responsibility for the married.

As for all those who are not married, we will not cease enjoining fidelity to the same moral beliefs. Our secularistic era may scoff at them as old-fashioned. But modernity and its worldly values do not abolish the continuing validity of St. Paul's words: "Your life is hidden with Christ in God. . . . Put to death then the parts of you that are earthly: immorality, impurity, passion, evil desire, and the greed that is idolatry" (Col. 3:3-5).

When one lives by faith, as all followers of Christ must, one is convinced that chastity and the refusal to engage in extra-marital sexual activity are the best protection against HIV-AIDS.

To our beloved Priests, Religious and other faithful who have committed themselves to a life of celibacy, we say: You are a sign for others that chastity lived for the Kingdom of God and a well integrated and ordered sexuality are not only possible but are actually being lived.

6. In the face of the rapidly spreading scourge of HIV-AIDS, we cannot overstate the need for a profound moral renewal of our people. This was the call of the Second Plenary Council of the Philippines for the transformation of our society (PCP-II, Acts and Decrees, e.g., no. 32). This too, is our call for the radical prevention of the HIV-AIDS disease. Nothing short of this can effectively respond to the deep-rooted moral cause of the problem. It is at depth a moral issue. We must not, therefore, forget the absolute imperative of moral renewal, while continuing the search for the medical solution.

Conclusion

We invite all persons of good will to be in solidarity with HIV-AIDS patients. They are our sisters and brothers. We see in their faces the suffering image of Jesus himself: What you do to the least of my brothers and sisters, you do it to me (cf., Mt. 25:40). As we minister to the afflicted, we proclaim to all the infinite compassion of God and the redeeming passion and death of Christ, the Savior of all.

May our Blessed Virgin Mary whom we invoke as Mother, "Health of the Sick" and "Comfort of the Afflicted" accompany us through this passion of modern times.

For and in the name of the
Catholic Bishops' Conference of the Philippines
(signed) Carmelo D. F. Morelos, D.D.
President
Setania Retreat House
Tagaytay City
January 23, 1993

Anti-Abortive Drugs Act of 1995

Tenth Congress of the Republic of the Philippines

First Regular Session
Senate, S.B. No. 1014
Introduced by Senator Tatad

Explanatory Note

Article II, Section 12 of the 1987 Constitution mandates the State to "protect the life of the mother and the life of the unborn from *conception.*" This particular provision makes our Constitution one of the few constitutions which, in the words of former Constitutional Commissioner and now Senator Blas Ople, has "a commitment to the protection of life, even in its incipient stage" as a "declaration of a commitment to a higher tone of our civilization."

However, eight years after the ratification of the Constitution, abortive drugs and devices continue to proliferate around the country and are even promoted actively by the Department of Health, the Commission on Population and various private population agencies in utter violation of the Constitution they are bound to uphold.

Of particular interest is the use of abortive drugs such as the Oral Contraceptives or what is commonly known as the "Pill." Some of these drugs have therapeutic value and may not therefore be banned outright. However, there is a need to regulate their use to prevent their wanton use for abortion purposes.

The continued use of abortive drugs to curb population growth despite the constitutional ban on abortion is based on the mistaken notion that these are merely contraceptives, that they do not terminate life but rather prevent its conception.

In an article published by the Human Life International, Bogomir M. Kuhar, Ph.D., president and founder of Pharmacists for Life, wrote that "oral contraceptives (one category of abortive drugs) rely on a tertiary abortifacient mechanism of preventing the implantation of a newly conceived baby." In particular, "low-dose oral contraceptives, due to their lesser amounts of active ingredients, permit more ovulation, more conception, and hence rely more heavily on chemical abortion as backup."

Another category of abortive drugs is Anti-Progesterones. This type includes the so-called "contraceptive vaccine." "Containing part of a hormone, human chorionic gonadotrophin (HCG), which is released by the ovum after fertilization and is necessary to maintain the pregnancy during the first six weeks, the vaccine creates antibodies to HCG and thereby prevents implantation."

Synthetic Prostaglandins, the third category of abortive drugs, "cause the most violent uterine contractions" and "are primarily used in second-trimester abortions from the 13th to the 22nd weeks of gestation."

Thus, the use of these and other abortive drugs, to the extent that they chemically terminate the life of a conceived child, clearly violates the pro-life dictates of the Constitution and the provision on the Rights of the Child (Article 3, (1)) of Presidential Decree No. 603, as amended, otherwise known as The Child and Youth Welfare Code, which states that "Every child is endowed with the dignity and worth of a human being from *the moment of his conception*, as generally accepted in medical parlance, and has, therefore, the right to be born well."

In view of the above, the bill enclosed seeks to regulate the use, production, sale, distribution or dispensation of abortive drugs, defining the same and providing penalties therefore. Passage of this bill is earnestly sought.

Francisco S. Tatad

AN ACT REGULATING THE USE, PRODUCTION, SALE, DISTRIBUTION OR DISPENSATION OF ABORTIVE DRUGS, DEFINING THE SAME, PROVIDING PENALTIES THEREFOR AND FOR OTHER PURPOSES.

Be it enacted by the Senate and House of Representatives of the Philippines in Congress assembled:

SECTION 1. This Act shall be known as the "Anti-Abortive Drugs Act of 1995."

SECTION 2. For the purpose of this Act, "Abortive Drug" shall be defined as any medicine, drug, chemical, or potion that acts or has the potential either to interfere with the implantation of the fertilized ovum onto the mother's womb or to interrupt pregnancy after implantation. It shall include but shall not be limited to such groups of abortive drugs as the Oral Contraceptives, Prostaglandins (not be confused with Prostaglandins with beneficial use) and Anti-progesterones.

SECTION 3. No abortive drug shall be sold, distributed or dispensed except through a prescription issued by a licensed physician.

SECTION 4. No physician shall prescribe any abortive drug for any person unless his physical or physiological condition justifies its use for therapeutic purposes.

SECTION 5. No woman shall use any abortive drug without the appropriate prescription from a qualified physician.

SECTION 6. All manufacturers of drugs shall label all abortive drugs or chemicals they produce indicating therein that such drugs have "abortifacient potential."

SECTION 7. The Department of Health shall serve as the implementing and monitoring agency for this Act. Within sixty (60) days from the approval of this Act, it shall formulate the implementing rules and guidelines necessary thereof, including measures that would guarantee the accurate and/or verifiable issuance, keeping and submission of prescriptions, records of purchases from drugstores, labeling of abortive drugs and such other measures as may be needed for the effective implementation of this Act.

SECTION 8. Violation of this Act shall be punishable by imprisonment of not less than six months and a fine not exceeding 5,000 pesos: *Provided*, that if the offender is a physician or practitioner, he shall suffer the additional penalty of the revocation of his license to practice his profession; *Provided, further*, that if the offender is a foreigner, he shall be deported without further proceedings after serving his sentence.

SECTION 9. This Act shall take effect upon its approval.

Approved.

The Patients' Rights Act of 1995

Tenth Congress of the Republic of the Philippines

First Regular Session
Senate S.B., No. 676
Introduced by Senator Webb

AN ACT DECLARING THE RIGHTS OF PATIENTS AND PRESCRIBING PENALTIES FOR VIOLATIONS THEREOF.

Be it enacted by the Senate and the House of Representatives of the Philippines in Congress assembled:

SECTION 1. *Short Title.* This Act shall be known as the "Patients' Rights Act of 1995."

SECTION 2. *Declaration of Policy.* The Philippine Constitution, in Section 1, Article XIII, states that the Congress shall give the highest priority to the enactment of measures that protect and enhance the right of all people to human dignity. Towards this end, it is hereby declared the policy of the State to ensure and protect the rights of patients to decent, humane, and quality health care.

SECTION 3. *Definition of Terms.* As used in this Act, the following terms are defined as follows:

(1) "Advance Directive"—a duly notarized document executed by a person of age and of sound mind, upon consultation with a physician and family members, which directs health care providers to refrain from providing prolonged life support when the situation arises that the person who executed such directive suffers a condition with little or no hope of reasonable recovery.

(2) "Communicable Disease"—an illness due to a specific infectious agent or its toxic products, arising through transmission of that agent or its products from reservoir to susceptible host, either directly as from an infected person or animal, or indirectly through the agency of an intermediate plant or animal host, a vector, or the inanimate environment.

(3) "Diagnostic Procedure"—any method used to establish the presence of the disease, and the nature and extent of such disease.

(4) "Emergency"—an unforeseen combination of circumstances which calls for immediate action to preserve the life of a person.

(5) "Health Care"—measures taken by a health care provider or that are taken in a health care institution in order to determine a patient's state of health or to restore or maintain it.

(6) "Health Care Institution"—a site devoted primarily to the maintenance and operation of facilities for the diagnosis, treatment, and care of individuals suffering from illness, disease, injury, or deformity, or in need of obstetrical or other medical and nursing care. It shall also be construed as any institution, building, or place where there are installed beds, or cribs, or bassinets for twenty-four hour use or longer by patients in the treatment of diseases, injuries, deformities, or abnormal physical and mental states, maternity cases or sanatorial care, or infirmaries, nurseries, dispensaries, and such other similar names by which they may be designated.

(7) "Health Care Professional"—any doctor, dentist, or other professional who is trained in heath care and duly licensed to practice in the Philippines.

(8) "Health Maintenance Organization"—an entity that provides, offers, or arranges for coverage of designated health services needed by plan members for a fixed prepaid premium.

(9) "Human Experimentation"—the physician's departure from standard medical practice of treatment for the purpose of obtaining new knowledge or testing a scientific hypothesis on human subjects.

(10) "Informed Consent"—the voluntary agreement of a person to undergo or be subjected to a procedure based on his understanding of the relevant consequences of receiving a particular treatment, as clearly explained by the health care provider. Such permission may be written, conveyed verbally, or expressed indirectly through an overt act.

(11) "Medically Necessary"—a service or procedure which is appropriate and consistent with diagnosis and which, using accepted standards of medical practice, could not be omitted without adversely affecting the patient's condition.

(12) "Patient"—a person who avails of health and medical care services or is otherwise the subject of such services.

(13) "Public Health and Safety"—the state of well-being of the population in general, the protection of which may require the curtailment or suspension of certain rights of patients.

(14)   "Serious Physical Injury"—a condition which, if left medically unattended, could lead to permanent disability.

(15)   "Treatment Procedure"—any scientifically accepted method used to remove the symptoms and cause of a disease.

SECTION 4. *The Rights of Patients*. The following rights of the patient shall be respected by all those involved in his care:

(1)   *Right to Medical Care and Treatment*

Every person has a right to health and medical care corresponding to his state of health, without any discrimination and within the limits of the resources available for health and medical care at the relevant time.

The patient has the right to health and medical care of good quality. In the course of such care, his human dignity, convictions and integrity shall be respected. His individual needs and culture shall be likewise respected.

If any person cannot immediately be given treatment that is medically necessary he shall, depending on his state of health, either be directed to wait for care, or be referred or sent for treatment elsewhere, where the appropriate care can be provided. If the patient has to wait for care, he shall be informed of the reason for the delay and the estimated waiting time.

Patients in emergency who are in danger of dying and/or who may have suffered serious physical injuries shall be extended immediate medical care and treatment without any deposit, pledge, mortgage or any form of advance payment for confinement or treatment

(2)   *Right to Informed Consent*

The patient has a right to a clear explanation, in layperson's terms, of all proposed procedures, whether diagnostic or therapeutic, including the identity of the person who will perform the said procedure, possibilities of any risk of mortality or serious side effects, problems related to recuperation, and probability of success, and he will not be subjected to any procedure without his informed consent: *Provided*, that in cases of emergency, when the patient is unconscious and/or incapable of giving consent and there is no one who can give consent in his behalf, then the physician can perform any diagnostic or treatment procedure as good practice of medicine dictates without such consent; *Provided further*, that when the law makes it compulsory for everyone to submit to a procedure, a consent is not necessary.

Informed consent shall be obtained from the patient concerned if he is of legal age and of sound mind, from the next of kin in case the patient is incapable of giving consent, or from the parents or legal guardian in the case of a minor or a mentally incapacitated individual, *Provided*, that if his parents or legal guardian refuses to give consent to a medical or surgical procedure necessary to save his life, the court upon petition of the physician or any person interested in the welfare of the child, may issue an order giving such consent.

The opinion of a minor patient concerning care or treatment measures shall be assessed, based on his age or level of development, and whenever possible, care shall be administered with his agreement.

(3)   *Right of Privacy*

The patient has a right to be left alone when this will not prejudice the provision of necessary medical care.

The patient has the right to be free from unwarranted publicity, except in the following cases: a) when his mental or physical condition is in controversy and the appropriate court in its discretion orders him to submit to a physical or mental examination by a physician; b) when public health and safety so demand; and c) when the patient waives this right.

(4)   *Right to Information*

The patient has a right to a clear, complete, and accurate evaluation of the nature and extent of his disease, the contemplated medical and surgical procedure and its probable outcome, economic costs, impact on lifestyle and work including side-effects and after-effects of the treatment, possible complications and other pertinent facts regarding his illness. However, if the disclosure of information to the patient will cause mental suffering and further impair his health, or cause the patient not to submit to medically necessary treatment, such disclosure may be withheld or deferred to some future opportune time, *Provided*, that his next of kin shall be consulted and given the relevant information.

The patient has the right to know the name and credentials of the physician responsible for his care or for coordinating such care. He may likewise request for similarly relevant information about any other health care provider directly involved in his care.

The patient has the right to examine and be given an itemized bill for services rendered in the facility or by his physician and other health care providers, regardless of the manner and source of payment. He is entitled to a thorough explanation of such bill should he find this incomprehensible.

The patient has a right to be informed by the physician or his delegate of his continuing health care requirements following discharge, including instructions about home medications, diet, physical activity and all other pertinent information to promote health and well-being.

(5) *Right of Privileged Communication*

The patient has the right to demand that all information, communication and records pertaining to his care be treated as confidential. A physician is not authorized to divulge any information to a third party who has no concern with the care and welfare of the patient, except: a) when such disclosure will benefit public health and safety; b) when it is in the interest of justice; and c) when the patient waives the confidential nature of such information.

Informing the spouse or the family to the first degree of the patient's medical condition shall not be considered a breach of confidentiality. Such disclosure shall be considered a fulfillment of the health care provider's duty to inform. In the case of a patient who has not reached the age of legal discretion or is mentally incapacitated, such information shall be given to the parents, legal guardian or his next of kin.

(6) *Right to Choose his Physician*

The patient is free to choose the physician to serve him except when a) he seeks medical treatment in a government hospital; b) he is confined in a charity ward; and c) he has entered into a contract with a health maintenance organization or any other health insurance organization which stipulates that the patient can only be served by a physician affiliated with the organization.

The patient has the right to discuss his condition with a consultant specialist, at the patient's request and expense. He also has the right to request, in cases of doubt, for a second opinion from another physician before agreeing to treatment, surgical operation or therapeutic procedure entailing a risk to health or life.

(7) *Right to Self-Determination*

The patient has the right to refuse diagnostic and treatment procedures, *Provided*, that a) he is of age and of sound mind; b) he is informed of the medical consequences of his refusal; c) he releases those involved in his care from any obligation relative to the consequences of his decision; and d) his refusal will not jeopardize public health and safety.

An adult with a sound mind may execute an advance directive for physicians not to put him on prolonged life support if, in the future, his condition is such that there is little or no hope of reasonable recovery. The qualifications listed as a, b, and c of the preceding paragraph shall be considered as satisfied if a patient whose condition makes him unable to express his will has executed an advance directive.

(8) *Right to Religious Belief*

The patient has the right to refuse medical treatment which may be contrary to his religious beliefs, subject to the limitations described in the preceding Subsection, *Provided*, that such a right shall not be imposed by parents upon their children who have not reached the age of legal discretion.

(9) *Right to Medical Records*

The patient is entitled to a summary of his medical history and condition which shall be accomplished by the attending physician. He has the right to view the contents of his medical record upon consultation with his attending physician. At his expense and within a reasonable period of time, he may obtain from the health care institution a reproduction of the same record, whether or not he has fully settled his financial obligations with the physician or institution concerned.

The health care institution shall issue a medical certificate, free of charge, to the patient upon discharge from the institution. Any other document that the patient may require for insurance claims shall also be made available to him within a reasonable period of time.

(10) *Right to Leave*

The patient has the right to leave a hospital or any other health care institution regardless of his physical condition, *Provided*, that the qualifications listed in the first paragraph of Subsection 7 hereof are satisfied.

No patient shall be detained against his will in any health care institution on the sole basis of his failure to fully settle his financial obligations with the physician or the health care institution, *Provided*, that he executes a promissory note covering the unpaid obligation, secured either by a mortgage or by the guarantee of a co-maker acceptable to the hospital or medical clinic who shall be jointly and solidarily liable with the patient for the unpaid obligation. Furthermore, when a patient dies, his relatives have the right to claim his cadaver subject to the condition stated herein.

(11) *Right to Refuse Participation in Medical Research*

The patient has the right to be advised if the health care provider plans to involve him in medical research, including but not limited to human experimentation that may affect his care or treatment. Such human experimentation may be performed only with the written informed consent of the patient.

(12) *Right to Correspondence and to Receive Visitors*
The patient has the right to communicate with relatives and other persons and to receive visitors subject to reasonable limits prescribed by the rules and regulations of the health care institution.

(13) *Right to Express Grievances*
The patient has the right to express complaints and grievances about the care and services received. The Secretary of Health, in consultation with health care providers, consumer groups and other concerned agencies, shall establish a grievance system wherein patients may seek redress of their grievances. Such a system shall afford all parties concerned with the opportunity to settle amicably all grievances. Any violation of the patients' rights enumerated in this Act shall constitute a valid ground for grievance.

(14) *Right to be Informed of His Rights and Obligations as a Patient*
Every person has the right to be informed of his rights and obligations as a patient. The Department of Health, in coordination with health care providers, professional and civic groups, the media, health insurance corporations, people's organizations, local government units, and other government agencies and non-governmental organizations, shall launch and sustain a nationwide information and education campaign to make known to people their rights as patients, as declared in this Act.

It shall be the duty of health care institutions to inform patients of their rights as well as of the institutions's rules and regulations that apply to the conduct of the patient while in the care of such an institution.

SECTION 5. *Penalties.* Any person found guilty of violating these rights shall be punished by a fine of not less than Ten Thousand Pesos (P10,000.00) but not more than Fifty Thousand Pesos (P50,000.00), and/or by imprisonment of not less than one year nor more than five years, or both by such fine and imprisonment, at the discretion of the court. Administrative sanctions, including the suspension or revocation of the violator's license to practice his profession, shall be imposed in addition to the penalties provided herein.

If the punishable act or omission is committed by an association, partnership, corporation or any other institution, its managing directors, partners, president, general manager, or other persons responsible for the offense shall be liable for the penalties provided for in this Act.

SECTION 6. *Rules and Regulations.* The Secretary of Health, in consultation with the Philippine Medical Association, the Philippine Hospital Association, and concerned private agencies, non-government organizations and people's organizations shall promulgate within 180 days from the effectivity of this Act such rules and regulations as may be necessary for its implementation.

The Implementing Rules and Regulations of this Act shall identify specific conditions under which the individual rights of patients, as stipulated in Subsections 3, 5, 7, and 8 of Section 4 hereof, may be curtailed or suspended in the interest of public health and safety.

SECTION 7. *Repealing Clause.* All acts, executive orders, administrative orders, rules and regulations, or parts thereof that are inconsistent with the provisions of this Act are hereby repealed or modified accordingly.

SECTION 8. *Effectivity.* This Act shall take effect fifteen (15) days after the date of its publication in at least two (2) major newspapers of national circulation.

Code of Ethics

Board of Medicine

ARTICLE I

GENERAL PROVISIONS

SECTION 1. The primary objectives of the practice of medicine is service to mankind irrespective of race, creed or political affiliation. In its practice, reward of financial gain should be a subordinate consideration.

SECTION 2. On entering his profession a physician assumes the obligation of maintaining the honorable tradition that confers upon him the well deserved title of "friend of man". He should cherish a proper pride in his calling, conduct himself as a gentleman, and endeavor to exalt the standards and extend the sphere of usefulness of his profession. He should adhere to the generally accepted principles of the International Code of Medical Ethics adopted by the Third General Assembly of the World Medical Association at London, England in October, 1949 as part of his professional conduct.

SECTION 3. In his relation to his patients, he shall serve their interests with the greatest solicitude, giving them always his best talent and skill.

SECTION 4. In his relation to the state and to the community, a physician should fulfill his civic duties as a good citizen, conform to the laws and endeavor to cooperate with the proper authorities in the due application of medical knowledge for the promotion of the common welfare.

SECTION 5. With respect to the relation of the physician to his colleagues, he should safeguard their legitimate interests, reputation, and dignity—bearing always in mind the golden rule "whatever ye would that man should do unto you, do you even so to them."

SECTION 6. The ethical principles actuating and governing a clinic or a group of physicians are exactly the same as those applicable to the individual physician. Specialties in the various fields of medical sciences are not exempt from the application of these principles.

ARTICLE II

DUTIES OF PHYSICIANS TO THEIR PATIENTS

SECTION 1. A physician should attend to his patients faithfully and conscientiously. He should secure for them all possible benefits that may depend upon his professional skill and care. As the sole tribunal to adjudge the physician's failure to fulfill his obligation to his patients is, in most cases, his own conscience, and violation of this rule on his part is discreditable and inexcusable.

SECTION 2. A physician is free to choose whom he will serve. He may refuse calls, or other medical services for reasons satisfactory to his professional conscience. He should, however, always respond to any request for his assistance in an emergency. Once he undertakes a case, he should not abandon nor neglect it. If for any reason he wants to be released from it, he should announce his desire previously, giving sufficient time or opportunity to the patient or his family to secure another medical attendant.

SECTION 3. In cases of emergency, wherein immediate action is necessary, a physician should administer at least first aid treatment and then refer the patient to a more qualified and competent physician if the case does not fall within his particular line.

SECTION 4. In serious cases which are difficult to diagnose and treat, or when the circumstances of the patient or the family so demand or justify, the attending physician should seek the assistance of his colleagues in consultation.

SECTION 5. A physician must exercise good faith and strict honesty in expressing his opinion as to the diagnosis, prognosis, and treatment of the cases under his care. Timely notice of the serious tendency of the disease should be given to the family or friends of the patients, and even to the patient himself if such information will serve the best interest of the patient and his family. It is highly unprofessional to conceal the gravity of the patient's condition, or to pretend to cure or alleviate a disease for the purpose of persuading the patient to take or continue the course of treatment, knowing that such assurance is without accepted basis. It is also unprofessional to exaggerate the condition of the patient.

SECTION 6. The medical practitioner should guard as a sacred trust anything that is confidential or private in nature that he may discover or that may be communicated to him in his professional relation with his patients, even after their death. He should never divulge this confidential information, or anything that may reflect upon the moral character of the person involved, except when it is required in the interest of justice, public health, or public safety.

SECTION 7. The medical profession not being a business and service being its primary concern, a physician should not charge exorbitant or excessive fees. In determining the amount of the fee, he should always consider the financial status of the patient, the nature of the case, the time consumed, his professional standing and skill and the average fees charged by physicians of the same standing in the same locality.

ARTICLE III

DUTIES OF PHYSICIANS TO THE COMMUNITY

SECTION 1. Physicians should cooperate with the proper authorities in the enforcement of sanitary laws and regulations and in the education of the people on matters relating to the promotion of the health of the individual as well as of the community. They should enlighten the public on the dangers of communicable diseases and other preventable diseases, and on all the measures for their prevention and cure, particularly in times of epidemic or public calamity. On such occasions, it is their duty to attend to the needs of the sufferers, even at the risk of their own lives and without regard to financial returns. At all times, it is the duty of the physician to notify the properly constituted public health authorities of every case of communicable disease under his care in accordance with the laws, rules and regulations of the health authorities of the Philippines.

SECTION 2. It is the duty of every physician, when called upon by the judicial authorities, to assist in the administration of justice on matters which are medico-legal in character.

SECTION 3. It is the duty of physicians to warn the public against the dangers and false pretensions of charlatans and quacks, since, their deceitful practice may cause injury to health and even loss of life.

SECTION 4. A physician should never cover up, help, aid or act as a dummy of any illegal practitioner, quack or charlatan.

SECTION 5. Solicitation of patients, directly or indirectly, through solicitors or agents, is unethical. Modest advertising may be allowed through professional cards, classified advertising, directories of signboard. In all these advertisements only the name, title, or profession, office hours and office and residence addresses should appear. In case of physicians specializing on a definitive branch of medicine, the specialty may be advertised by stating "Practice limited to (specialty)," "Ophthalmologist," etc. Advertising and publishing personal superiority, possession of special certificates or diplomas, postgraduate training abroad, specific methods of treatments or operative techniques or advertising former connection with hospitals or clinics are likewise unethical. Guaranteeing or warranting treatments or operations is objectionable.

SECTION 6. No physician should advertise through the radio, television or movies nor allow the publication of reports or comments on cases or methods of treatment in any newspaper or magazine. Only medical articles which will contribute to the knowledge and education of the public on general health matters may be published and the author may be identified provided the article is neither self-laudatory nor in any way related to his clinical practice. In case any picture or a laudatory article is published by anybody without the consent or knowledge of the physician concerned, the latter should make a written protest and disclaimer where the original article in question was published. A copy of this letter should also be furnished to the component society to whom the physician belongs and to the PMA Secretariat.

SECTION 7. The physician-columnist must be well informed and up-to-date in the subject matter of his column. The scope of the medical column should be in the form of general information, of educational value and of public interest, such as needs for yearly periodic consultations, preventive measures, formation of good health habits, explanation of need for diagnostic sides, emergency measures, and other topics of general interest to the health of the public. Medical columns should not make specific diagnosis or therapy or be projected to individual cases. The physician-columnist should not be in active clinical practice. If, however, the physician-columnist is in active clinical practice, his authorship must be in the form of a pseudonym or the columns may be published under the sponsorship of a medical society or a specialty society to which he belongs.

SECTION 8. Humanity requires every physician to render his services gratuitously to poor and indigent persons who are in need of his attendance. The endowed institution and organization for mutual benefit or for accident, sickness or life insurance or for analogous purposes have no claim upon physicians for unremunerated service.

ARTICLE IV
DUTIES OF PHYSICIANS TO THEIR COLLEAGUES AND TO
THE PROFESSION

SECTION 1. Physicians should labor together in harmony, each giving freely to others whatever advantage he may have to contribute.

SECTION 2. A physician should willingly render gratuitous service to a colleague, to his wife and minor children or even to his father or mother provided the latter are aged and are being supported by the colleague. He should, however, be furnished the necessary traveling expenses and compensated for all medicines and supplies necessary in the treatment of the patient. This provision shall not apply to physicians who are no longer in practice nor to physicians who are engaged only or purely in business.

SECTION 3. In difficult and serious cases or in those which are outside the competence of the attending physician, he should always suggest and ask consultation. Only experienced physicians who are senior to the attending physician or who have had special training and experience in a particular line of medicine should be selected by the latter as consultants.

SECTION 4. Out of consideration for the object of consultation and for the physician's duty to uphold the honor and dignity of his profession, no physician should meet in consultation with anyone who is not qualified by law to practice medicine. In arranging for a consultation the attending physician should fix the hours of the meeting. However, it is his duty to make the appointment in a way satisfactory to the consultant.

SECTION 5. Every physician participating in a consultation should endeavor to observe punctuality. Unless the cause of delay is known, if the attending physician does not arrive within a reasonable time after the appointed hour, the consultant should, according to the circumstances attending the case, be at liberty either to regard the consultation as postponed or to see the patient alone. In the latter case, he should leave his conclusions in writing in a sealed envelope. On the other hand, if the consultant does not appear at the fixed time, the attending physician, after a reasonable period of waiting, and with the consent of the patient, or his family, may either arrange for another consultation or give permission for the consultant to examine the patient and forward to him a written statement of his opinion. In giving such written opinion, the consultant must see to it that the opinion is under seal and that his statements are courteously worded.

SECTION 6. The attending physician should give the consultant all necessary information relating to the case. This should be done in a place away from the patient and his family. After this the consultant should be brought in and introduced to the patient by the attending physician, who may examine the patient again, if he thinks it necessary to note any possible changes before turning his patient over to the consultant. The latter then should proceed to make a thorough examination. During the examination, the attending physician may make patient remarks or observation. While in the presence of the patient or of his family, the consultant should not make any remarks about the diagnosis, etiology, prognosis, or treatment or hint of any possible error of the attending physician.

SECTION 7. In a secluded place away from the patient the physicians should discuss the case and determine the course of treatment to be followed. Neither statement nor discussion of the case should take place before the patient or his family or friends, not only to save the attending physician from possible embarrassment, but also to prevent all possible misapprehension which susceptive lay persons might easily derive from the plain discussion usually unavoidable in such cases.

SECTION 8. Once the discussion is terminated, the result of the deliberations should be announced. The duty of announcing it to the patient's family or friends should be mutually arranged between the attending physician and the consultant, and no opinion or information should be announced without previous deliberation and concurrence.

SECTION 9. Differences of opinion should not be divulged; but when there is an irreconcilable disagreement, the circumstances should be frankly, courteously, and impartially explained to the patient's family or friends.

SECTION 10. When a consultation is over and the physician in charge is designated, the latter shall be responsible for the care and treatment of the patient. He may, however, suggest calling in any other physician whom he regards as competent to help or to advise. He may at anytime change or abandon the course of treatment outlined and agreed upon at the consultation, if and when, in his opinion, such action is required by the condition of the patient. If he does this, he should at the next consultation state his reasons for departing from the course previously agreed upon because it is his duty to follow the treatment outlined and refrain from changing it for trivial motives. If an emergency occurs and the physician in charge is not available, the consultant should attend to the case until the arrival of his colleague, but should not take further charge of it except with the consent of the attending physician.

SECTION 11. Cases which appear to be out of the proper line of practice of the physician in charge or refractory in spite of the usual clinical treatment, or with a grave prognosis should be referred to those who specialize in that class of ailments. It is desirable that the patient brings with him a letter of introduction giving the history of the case, its diagnosis and treatment, and all the details that may be of service to the specialist. The latter should, in turn, reply in writing to the physician in charge, giving his opinion of the case together with the course of treatment he recommends. These opinions or suggestions must be regarded as strictly confidential.

SECTION 12. A physician should observe utmost caution, tact and prudence, both in words and in action, as regards the professional conduct of another physician, particularly when it concerns a patient previously treated by the latter or actually under his care. In his dealings with patients not under his care, he should not say or do anything that might lessen the patient's confidence reposed in the attending physician.

SECTION 13. Whenever a physician is compelled to make a social or business call on a patient under the professional case of another physician, he should not make inquiries or comments as to the etiology, diagnosis, treatment, or prognosis of the case. The most that may be mentioned is the general condition of the patient or other topics foreign to the case.

SECTION 14. A physician should not take charge of or prescribe for a patient already under the care of another physician, unless the case is one of emergency, or the physician in attendance has relinquished the case, or the services of the attending physician has been dispensed with.

SECTION 15. A physician should never examine or treat a hospitalized patient of another without the latter's knowledge and consent except in cases of emergency, but in the latter instance, the physician should not continue the treatment but return the patient to his attending physician after the emergency has passed.

SECTION 16. A physician called upon to attend a patient of another physician either because of an emergency, or because the family physician asks for it, or is not available should attend only to the patient's immediate needs. His attendance ceases when the emergency is over or on the arrival of the physician in charge after he has reported the condition found and treatment administered; and he should not charge the patient for his services without the knowledge of the attending physician.

SECTION 17. Whenever in the absence of the family physician several physicians have been simultaneously called in an emergency case because of the alarm and anxiety of the family or friends, the first to arrive should be considered as physician in charge, unless the patient or his family has special preference for some other one among those who are present. As a matter of courtesy, the acting physician in charge should request, at the start, that the family physician be called. When the patient is taken to the hospital, the attending physician of the hospital, likewise should communicate with the family physician so as to give him the option of attending the case.

SECTION 18. Public interest demands that the relation between government and private physicians should be friendly and cordial for the promotion and protection of public health depend greatly upon the cooperation of government and private physicians.

SECTION 19. The physician should carefully refrain from making unfair and unwarranted criticism of other physicians, and, even in justified circumstances, criticism should be made in a constructive way and only directly and privately to the physicians involved. Whenever there is an irreconcilable difference of opinion, or conflict of interest between physicians, which cannot be adjusted by both sides alone, the matter should be referred to a committee of impartial physicians or other competent bodies for arbitration.

SECTION 20. When a physician is requested by a colleague to take care of a patient during his temporary absence or when because of an emergency he is asked to see the patient of a colleague, the physician should treat the patient in the same manner and with the same delicacy as he would have wanted his own patient cared for under similar conditions. The patient should be returned to the care of the attending as soon as possible.

SECTION 21. When a physician attends a woman in labor in the absence of another who has been engaged to attend, such physician should relinquish the patient to the one first engaged upon his arrival. The physician is entitled to compensation for the professional services he may have rendered.

SECTION 22. A true physician does not base his practice on exclusive dogma or sectarian systems, for medicine is a liberal profession. It has no creed, no party, no master. Neither is subject to any bond except that of truth. A physician should keep abreast of the advancement of medical science; contribute to its progress; and associate with his colleagues in any of the recognized medical societies, so that he may broaden his horizon through the exchange of ideas, and in order that he may contribute his time, energy, and means towards making these societies represent the ideas of the profession. The medical journal is one of the most important instruments through which these objectives may be accomplished. It is therefore necessary that editors and members of editorial boards of medical journals should possess adequate qualifications. And to the end in view all editors and members of the editorial boards of national medical journals will be recommended by the Philippine Association of Medical Writers, Inc. to the Executive Council, and in case of specialty and component medical society journals, the appointment of editors and members of editorial boards will be left at the discretion of their respective affiliate specialty or component medical societies concerned. Furthermore, the contents of medical journals should conform to accepted standards as provided for by the Philippine Association of Medical Writers, Inc.

SECTION 23. A physician should be upright, diligent, sober, modest, and well-versed in both the science and the art of his profession. Extravagance, intemperance, and superstitions are most destructive to the professional reputation, influence, and confidence; and they are not only financially but also morally disastrous.

SECTION 24. Advertising by means of untruthful or unprovable statements in newspapers or other publications, or exaggerated announcements on shingles and signboards, calculated to mislead or deceive the public, or made in a manner not consistent with good moral and right professional dealings with a patient, is unprofessional. Announcements in newspapers, or in signboards or shingles, should be restricted to the facts about the location of clinics, office hours, and limitation of practice. It is equally incompatible with honorable standing in the profession to solicit patients by circulars, by advertisements, or by personal relations to procure patients indirectly through solicitors or agents.

SECTION 25. It is unprofessional for a physician to help or to employ unqualified persons for the purpose of evading the legal restriction governing the practice of medicine.

SECTION 26. It is degrading to the good name of the medical profession to prescribe, dispense or manufacture secret remedies or to promote their use in any way. It is likewise unprofessional to promise or boast of radical cures or to exhibit publicly testimonial of success in the treatment of diseases.

SECTION 27. It is degrading to the professional character for physicians deliberately to prolong the progress of treatment of diseases for questionable motives, or to establish an unjust competition among physicians in the community by unwarranted lowering of fees.

SECTION 28. When a patient is referred by one physician to another for consultation or for treatment whether the physician in charge accompanies the patient or not, it is unprofessional to give or to receive commission by whatever term it may be called or under any guise or pretext whatsoever. It is unprofessional for a physician to pay or offer to pay, or to receive or solicit commission for the purpose of gaining patients or for recommending professional service.

SECTION 29. Physicians should expose without fear or favor, before the proper medical or legal tribunals corrupt or dishonest conduct of members of the profession. All questions affecting the professional reputation of a member or members of the medical society should be considered only before proper medical tribunals, in executive sessions or by special or duly appointed committees on ethical relations. Every physician should aid in safeguarding the profession against the admission to its ranks of those who are unfit or unqualified because of deficiency in moral character or education.

ARTICLE V
DUTIES OF PHYSICIANS TO ALLIED PROFESSIONALS

SECTION 1. Physicians should cooperate with and safeguard the interest, reputation, and dignity of every pharmacist, dentist, and nurse, because all of them have as their objective the amelioration of human suffering. But, should they violate their respective professional ethics, they thereby forfeit all claims to favorable considerations of the public and of physicians.

SECTION 2. Physicians should never sign or allow to be published any testimonial certifying the efficacy value and superiority and recommending the use of any drug, medicine, food product, instrument or appliance or any other object or product related to their practice specialty when published in a lay newspaper or magazine or broadcast through the radio or television. When such testimonials are published or broadcast without his knowledge and consent, he should immediately make the necessary rectification and order the discontinuance thereof.

SECTION 3. A physician should neither pay commissions to any person who refers cases to or help him in acquiring patients nor receive commission from druggists, laboratory men, radiologists or other co-workers in the diagnosis and treatment of patients for referring patients to them.

ARTICLE VI
AMENDMENTS

SECTION 1. The House of Delegates of the Philippine Medical Association, upon recommendation of the Executive Council, by a majority vote of all the delegates may amend or repeal this Code or adopt a new Code of Ethics of the

Medical Profession in the Philippines. Any amendment shall be a part of this Code of Medical Ethics and such amendments shall become effective after thirty (30) days following the completion of its publication in the *Official Gazette*.

ARTICLE VII
PENAL PROVISIONS

SECTION 1. The Code of Ethics shall be published in the *Official Gazette* to have the force and effect of law. Copies of this Code shall be distributed every year to all physicians during their Annual Conventions and published once a year in all medical journals published in the Philippines for the proper information and guidance of all physicians both in private practice and in the government service and shall also be distributed among all new physicians immediately following their oath taking. It shall be included in the curriculum of all medical schools as part of the course of study of legal medicine, ethics and medical jurisprudence.

SECTION 2. Violation of any one of the provisions of this Code of Ethics shall constitute unethical and unprofessional conduct and therefore a sufficient ground for the reprimand, suspension or revocation of the certificate of registration of the offending physician in accordance with the provisions of Section 24, paragraph (12) of the Medical Act of 1959, Republic Act 2382.

The Philippines

Angeles Tan Alora and Josephine M. Lumitao

The Philippine archipelago comprises 7,107 islands (800 of which are inhabited) lying between the South China Sea and the Pacific Ocean. It comprises a land area of approximately 300,000 square kilometers; it spans 1,854 kilometers from north to south and has a coastline of approximately 34,536 kilometers. The Philippines is divided geographically and culturally into 14 regions (12 Christian and 2 autonomous non-Christian). There are 73 provinces, 60 cities, 1,537 municipalities, and 41,292 *barangays*. Manila is the capital of the Philippines. Metropolitan Manila is the seat of administration, culture, art, education, commerce, and industry.

Filipinos are basically of Malay stock, with a sprinkling of Chinese, American, Spanish, and Arab blood. A long history of Western colonial rule, interspersed with the visits of merchants and traders, has evolved a people with a unique blend of East and West in appearance and culture.

In 1990, the population was 60,697,994; 48.7 percent lived in urban areas, and 51.3 percent lived in rural areas. The median age was 19 years; 39.5 percent were 3 years of age or younger, and the dependency ratio (0–14 years and more than 65 years divided by 15–64 years) was 75.3. In 1995, the population was 68,614,162 million. The growth rate was 2.32 percent.

Approximately 83 percent of the population is Catholic, 5 percent Muslim (mainly Mindanao); 5 percent belong to two Philippine independent churches, and the remainder belong primarily to smaller Christian denominations and Buddhism.

Filipino is the country's official language, but 111 dialects are spoken. English is taught in schools and widely used in business. Approximately 70 percent of Filipinos speak English. Approximately 93 percent of Filipinos older than 10 years of age can read and write.

The 1996 gross national product (GNP) was P8.4 (in million pesos). The GNP per capita (1992) was P12,234. The average household income (1991) was P89,571 in urban areas and P41,199 in rural areas. Of the total labor force of more than 28 million in 1995, 25.7 million were employed and 2.3 million were unemployed; thus, the unemployment rate was approximately 9 percent.

In 1996, 2.8 percent of sectoral expenditures (P11.47 billion) was allocated for health. The 1991 average annual family expenditure for health was P180 (1.8

percent of income). In 1995, there were 1,700 hospitals with a bed capacity of 80,000 (53 percent belonging to the government). In 1994 the numbers of government medical practitioners were as follows: 4,574,000 physicians, 1,997,000 dentists, 4,917,000 registered nurses, and 11,187,000 midwives.

Poverty threshold in 1994	P8885
Poverty incidence	40.6 percent
Population in 1996	70.1 million

Tables 1 through 6 provide additional data.

Table 1. AIDS in the Philippines

Reported Modes of Transmission	Cumulative Totals 1984– June 1997		1994		1995		1996		1997 (Jan–June)	
	HIV+	AIDS	HIV+	AIDS	HIV+	AIDS	HIV+	AIDS	HIV+	AIDS
Heterosexual contact	476	162	61	30	55	29	80	26	37	7
Homosexual contact	146	82	20	14	21	13	29	13	13	5
Bisexual contact	46	28	3	0	9	6	7	2	4	1
Blood/blood products	11	9	4	4	1	0	1	1	0	0
Injecting drug use	5	2	0	1	1	1	2	1	0	0
Needle prick injuries	2	1	0	0	0	0	1	0	0	0
Perinatal	12	5	2	1	0	0	3	2	1	0
No exposure reported	218	21	30	4	30	3	33	6	0	0
Total	916	310	119	56	117	52	156	51	55	13

Source: AIDS Registry.

Table 2. Mortality: Ten Leading Causes (number, crude death rate per 100,000 population, percentage of total deaths), 1986–1990 and 1991 (5-year average)

Cause	1986–1990			1991		
	No.	*Rate*	*Percentage of Total Deaths*	*No.*	*Rate*	*Percentage of Total Deaths*
Pneumonias	47,655	81.0	14.6	36,705	57.7	12.3
Diseases of the heart	41,939	71.3	12.9	46,381	72.9	15.6
Tuberculosis, all forms	27,386	46.5	8.4	22,814	35.9	7.7
Diseases of the vascular system	31,647	53.8	9.7	32,981	51.8	11.1
Malignant neoplasms	20,812	35.4	6.4	22,384	35.2	7.5
Diarrheas	9,512	16.2	2.9	5,497	8.6	1.8
Accidents	11,438	19.4	3.5	10,961	17.2	3.7
Septicemia	4,868	8.3	1.5	5,992	9.4	2.0
Respiratory conditions of fetus and newborn	6,478	11.0	2.0	4,973	7.8	1.7
Nephritis, nephrotic syndrome, and neprosis	5,123	8.7	1.6	5,024	7.9	1.7

Source: Health Intelligence Services, Department of Health.

Table 3. Mortality: Ten Leading Causes (number, crude death rate per 100,000 population, and percentage of total deaths), 1987–1991 and 1992 (5-year average)

Cause	1987–1991			1992		
	No.	*Rate*	*Percentage of Total Deaths*	*No.*	*Rate*	*Percentage of Total Deaths*
Pneumonias	44,871	74.3	14.0	42,074	64.4	13.2
Diseases of the heart	43,383	71.9	13.6	49,022	75.0	15.3
Tuberculosis, all forms	25,828	42.8	8.1	23,356	35.7	7.3
Diseases of the vascular system	32,363	53.6	10.1	35,414	54.2	11.1
Malignant neoplasms	21,609	35.8	6.8	23,946	36.6	7.5
Diarrheas	8,443	14.0	2.6	6,742	10.3	2.1
Accidents	11,560	19.1	3.6	11,292	17.3	3.5
Septicemia	5,160	8.5	1.6	5,774	8.9	1.8
Other diseases of the respiratory system	6,511	10.8	2.0	6,967	10.7	2.2
Chronic obstructive pulmonary diseases and allied conditions	7,521	12.5	2.4	9,391	14.4	2.9

Source: Health Intelligence Services, Department of Health.

Table 4.   Life Expectancy at Birth in the Philippines, 1960 to 2030 (in years)

Year	Both Sexes	Male	Female
1960[a]	53.1	51.2	55.0
1970[b]	55.7	54.2	57.2
1975	58.4	56.9	59.9
1980[c]	61.6	59.8	63.4
1981	61.9	60.1	63.7
1982	62.2	60.4	64.0
1983	62.5	60.7	64.3
1984	62.8	61.0	64.6
1985	63.1	61.3	64.9
1986	63.4	61.6	65.2
1987	63.7	61.9	65.5
1988	64.0	62.2	65.8
1989	64.3	62.5	66.1
1990	64.6	62.8	66.4
1995	66.1	64.4	67.8
2000	67.6	66.0	69.2
2010	70.3	68.8	71.8
2020	72.4	71.2	73.6
2030	73.6	72.8	74.4

[a]Reproduced from Wilfredo L. Reyes, "Philippine Population Growth and Heath Development," in *First Conference on Population, 1965* (Quezon City: University of the Philippines Press, 1966), 246.

[b]Starting in 1970, data are from National Statistics and Inter-Agency Committee on Population and Vital Statistics, "Revised Population Projections for the Philippines and Its Regions, 1980–2030," presented at 6th National Population Welfare Congress, 17 November 1983.

[c]Starting in 1980, estimates are from Moderate Mortality Decline Assumption National Statistics Office.

Table 5.   Population of the Philippines, 1799–1995

Year	Population	Average Annual Rate of Increase	Source of Data
1799	1,502,574		Fr. Buzeta
1800	1,561,251	3.91	Fr. Zuniga
1812	1,933,331	1.80	Cedulas
1819	2,106,230	1.23	Cedulas
1829	2,593,287	2.10	Church
1840	3,096,031	1.62	Local officials
1850	3,857,424	2.22	Fr. Buzeta
1858	4,290,381	1.34	Bowring
1870	4,712,006	0.78	Guia de Manila
1877	5,567,685	2.41	Census
1887	5,984,727	0.72	Census
1896	6,261,339	0.50	Prof. Plehn's estimate (based on census records)
1903	7,635,426	2.87	Census
1918	10,314,310	2.03	Census
1939	16,000,303	2.11	Census
1948	19,234,182	2.07	Census
1960	27,087,685	2.89	Census
1970	36,684,486	3.08	Census
1975	42,070,660	2.78	Census
1980	48,098,460	2.71	Census
1990	60,703,206[a]	2.35	Census
1995	68,614,162	2.32	Census

Note: Population from 1799 to 1896 excludes non-Christians.

[a]Includes household population, homeless population, Filipinos in Philippine embassies/
consulates and missions abroad, and Filipinos living in institutional living quarters such as penal
institutions, orphanages, hospitals, military camps, etc., at time of census.

Source: National Statistics Office.

Table 6.   Total Number of Families, Total and Average Family Income, and
Expenditures by Income Class, Urban and Rural, 1991

| | | Income | | Expenditures | |
Income Class	Total No. of Families (thousands)	Total (thousands of pesos)	Average (pesos)	Total (thousands of pesos)	Average (pesos)
URBAN					
Total	5,938	531,919,567	89,571	418,971,428	70,551
Under P10,000	85	625,877	7,403	852,786	10,086
10,000–19,999	402	6,332,940	15,753	6,729,394	16,740
20,000–29,999	643	16,195,551	25,172	15,824,940	24,596
30,000–39,999	689	24,126,630	35,010	22,294,314	32,351
40,000–49,999	617	27,703,508	44,891	25,162,603	40,774
50,000–59,999	570	31,250,558	54,851	27,888,251	48,950
60,000–79,999	824	57,098,235	69,314	48,973,305	60,665
80,000–99,999	550	49,280,885	89,689	41,689,725	75,873
100,000–149,000	792	96,203,691	121,540	77,143,370	97,460
150,000–249,000	505	94,934,472	188,147	72,820,235	144,319
250,000–499,000	207	67,881,568	327,935	51,371,544	248,175
500,000+	56	60,285,652	1,071,488	27,220,961	483,812
RURAL					
Total	6,037	248,712,904	41,199	203,644,774	33,733
Under P10,000	222	1,698,924	7,656	2,044,998	9,216
10,000–19,999	1,246	19,359,093	15,543	19,809,931	15,905
20,000–29,999	1,502	37,177,119	24,749	35,122,803	23,382
30,000–39,999	1,043	36,018,191	34,546	31,491,159	30,204
40,000–49,999	634	28,243,152	44,563	23,714,128	37,417
50,000–59,999	409	22,306,927	54,545	17,664,217	43,192
60,000–79,999	411	28,103,492	68,441	22,104,103	53,830
80,000–99,999	223	19,710,095	88,393	14,862,554	66,654
100,000–149,000	226	26,878,313	119,212	19,375,849	85,936
150,000–249,000	89	16,627,863	187,102	11,321,248	127,390
250,000–499,000	30	9,372,300	309,576	5,070,241	167,475
500,000+	4	3,217,434	860,024	1,063,544	284,287

Note: Final results of the 1988 Family Income and Expenditure Survey (FIES) exclude data for
Rizal province because fire destroyed completed questionnaires from this province.

Sources: 1985, 1988, and 1991, FIES, National Statistics Office; 1996, Philippine Statistical Yearbook, National Statistics Coordination Board.

Glossary

Awa compassion

Barkada peer group

Budhi conscience, the locus of moral decisions

Hilot traditional birth assistant

Hiya a painful emotion that arises from a relationship with an authority figure that inhibits self-assertion in situations perceived as dangerous to one's
ego. Embarrassment, shyness, timidity.

Kababang Loob humility

Kabutihan goodness

Kalooban the will

Lagay a tip to avoid delay

Lakad an attempt to smooth out difficulties by using a network of personal
connections

Lusot an escape from a difficult situation as painlessly as possible

Malasakit care

Nakakahiya a hesitancy because of propriety or good manners

Napahiya shame, guilt

Pakikisama a seeking of harmony with others

Palusot an excuse

Utang Na Loob a debt of gratitude

Walang Budhi a person without a conscience

Walang Hiya an absence of the *hiya* inhibition

Walang Utang Na Loob an absence of gratitude

Contributors

Angles Tan Alora, M.D., M.A.Ed., Dean, Faculty of Medicine and Surgery, Department of Medicine, University of Santo Tomas, Manila, the Philippines

Antonio Cabezon, O.P., S.T.D., Professor of Moral Theology and Bioethics, University of Santo Tomas, Manila, the Philippines

H. Tristram Engelhardt, Jr., Ph.D., M.D., Professor, Center for Medical Ethics and Health Policy, Baylor College of Medicine; and Professor, Department of Philosophy, Rice University, Houston, Texas, U.S.A.

Angelica Francisco, M.D., Assistant Professor, Department of Bioethics, De la Salle University, Health Sciences Campus, Dasmarinas, Cavite, the Philippines

Letty Gurdiel Kuan, Ph.D., R.N., Professor, College of Nursing, University of The Philippines, Manila, the Philippines

Rev. Tamerlane Recuenco Lana, O.P., S.T.D., Office of the Rector, University of Santo Tomas, University of Santo Tomas, Manila, the Philippines

Most Rev. Leonardo Z. Legaspi, O.P., D.D., Archbishop of Nueva Caceres, Director of Bioethics Office, Catholic Bishops' Conference of the Philippines

Josephine Lumitao, M.D., Professor, Department of Anatomy and Bioethics, Faculty of Medicine and Surgery, University of Santo Tomas, Manila, the Philippines

Edna G. Monzon, M.D., Department of Medicine, Faculty of Medicine and Surgery, University of Santo Tomas; and Philippine Heart Center for Asia, Manila, the Philippines

Edmund D. Pellegrino, M.D., Director, Center for Clinical Bioethics, and John Carroll Professor of Medicine and Medical Ethics, Georgetown University Medical Center, Washington, D.C., U.S.A.

Victoria Pusung, College of Nursing, University of Santo Tomas, Manila, the Philippines

Rev. Danilo C. Tiong, S.T.L., chair, Department of Bioethics, De la Salle University, Health Sciences Campus, Dasmarinas, Cavite, the Philippines

Mary Jean Villareal-Guno, M.D., Department of Pediatrics, Faculty of Medicine and Surgery, University of Santo Tomas, and Training Office, Santo Tomas University Hospital, Manila, the Philippines

Index

abortion, viii, 35, 36, 59, 106
advance directive, 133, 137–38
AIDS (Acquired Immune Deficiency
    Syndrome), 81–88, 125–29, 152.t1
allocation of resources, viii, 13, 18, 30, 32, 34,
    36, 39, 67, 69, 70, 76, 77, 79, 81–82, 85, 87, 97,
    103–07, 112, 116, 117–18, 122, 135
Amundsen, D., 67
Andres, T. D., 4, 23, 76
Angeles, R. R., 116
Anti-Abortive Drugs Act of 1995, 130–32
Antonio, Jr., Dr. Domingo, 116–18
Appelbaum, P. S., 48
Ashley, B., 83, 92
Atkinson, A., 115
autonomy, v, vii, 3, 14–15, 24–29, 42, 59, 63, 77,
    94, 96–98
awa, 55; definition, 157

bahala na, 13, 16, 76. *See also* fatalism
Barclay, W. R., 77
barkada, 31–32, 83, 95; definition, 157
Beauchamp, T., 4, 93
beneficence, 15, 59, 70
bioethics, v, vii–viii, xi–xiv, 3–22, 27–28, 36, 43,
    48, 57, 59, 61, 63, 66, 95–96, 98, 106, 108;
    Code of Ethics, 141–49
birth control, 30–39, 52. *See also* Catholicism
Bonifacio, M. F., 9, 11
Brisker, E. M., 50
Brodeur, D., 92
Brody, B., 78
budhi, 55; definition, 157. *See also walang budhi*
Bulatao, J., 8, 9

Catholicism, viii, 6–7, 13, 48, 75, 85–86, 95, 97,
    151; and conscience, 52–60; and family
    planning and contraception, 30–31, 33–35,
    36–38, 83; hospitals, 34, 75–77, 106, 112–13;
    and organ transplantation, 89–93. *See also*
    Second Vatican Council
cheating (in medical school), viii, 61–66
Childress, J., 93
Church, A. T., 4
confidentiality, 4, 15, 23–29, 81–82, 84, 86, 87,
    96, 137, 142, 146. *See also* privacy, patient's
    right to
Connelly, J. E., 50
conscience, 35–36, 48, 52–60. *See also budhi*

contraception. *See* birth control
cooperation, formal, 57–59; material, 57–59

Davis, H., 58
death, 14, 16–17, 48, 56, 75–78, 85, 86, 89,
    94–102, 109, 117, 119, 126, 128, 142. *See also*
    mortality rates in Philippines
decision making, vii, 8, 9, 14–17, 23–24, 36, 38,
    42–43, 63, 65, 67, 75–77, 79, 82, 85, 87, 95–99,
    103. *See also* allocation of resources;
    conscience
disclosure of information, 49, 62, 85, 87, 136–37
Drane, J., 6
drugs, 64–66, 85–86, 106; abortifacient, 132;
    cost, 50, 114; dumping, 99–121; generic,
    112–18; overprescribing, 114; trials, 108–11.
    See also abortion; Generics Act;
    pharmaceutical industry
dumping, 119–24
Dwyer, J. M., 84
dying. *See* death

Engelhardt, Jr., H. T., v, vii, ix–x, xi–xiv, 5, 78
euthanasia, 95, 97
extraordinary treatment, 95, 97; withdrawal
    of, 97

Faden, R., 48
Fallermurn, S., 50
family planning. *See* birth control
family, 3–22, 23–46. *See also* birth control
fatalism, 7, 10, 13, 85, 87, 91, 94, 97–98. See also
    bahala na
futility of medical treatments, 85

Generics Act, 113–16. *See also* drugs
Gorospe, V. R., 4, 68, 76

Haring, B., 92
Harvey, J. C., 90
health maintence organization (HMO), 105
hilot, 104–05; definition, 157. *See also* traditional
    birth assistant (TBA)
HIV (Human Immunodeficiency Virus),
    81–88, 125–29, 152.t1
hiya, 7, 10–11, 15–17, 36, 47, 55, 104, 109;
    definition, 157
honesty, 8, 61–66, 142
Horan, J. K., 49
Hoshino, K., 6, 15

hospitals, 16, 18, 34, 36, 48, 49, 58, 77–79, 82–85, 89, 96, 103, 104–06, 108, 112–13, 116–18, 121–22, 138, 143, 152; right to treatment in a government, 137. *See also* Catholicism
Human Life International, 130

individualism, xiii, 8; vs. family, *see* family
informed consent, vii, 15–17, 23–29, 94, 108, 109–10, 134, 135–36, 138
insurance, medical or health, 78, 105, 137, 138, 139, 144
Islam, 3, 7. *See also* Muslim

justice, v, 8, 9, 13, 15, 50, 53, 67–68, 80, 90, 93, 104, 122, 137,142–43

kababang loob, 47; definition, 157
kabutihan, 55; definition, 157
kalooban, 55; definition, 157
Koch, A., 58
Kuan, L. G., 24, 40
Kuhar, B. M., 130–31

lagay, 7, 10, 14, 18; definition, 157
lakad, 7, 10, 14, 18; definition, 157
life expectancy in Philippines, 154.t4
lusot, 7, 10, 14, 18, 64, 104, 109, 110; definition, 157

malasakit, 55; definition, 157
Mazur, D. J., 48
McCormick, R., 78
medical ethics. *See* bioethics
Mendez, P. P., 23
Mertz, D., 81
Miles, S., 84
Miranda, D., 67, 76, 114
Miranda, F. E., 13
Morreim, E. H., 50
mortality rates in Philippines, 153.t2 & 3. *See also* death
Muslim, 7, 13, 151. *See also* Islam

nakakahiya, 10–11; definition, 157
napahiya, 10–11; definition, 157
natural family planning. *See* birth control
Nelson, H., 69
Nelson, J., 69
nepotism, viii, 10, 67–74
non-maleficence, 15
O'Donnell, T. J., 92
organ transplantation, 89–93, 116–18
O'Rourke, K., 83, 92

Paguio, W. C., 4
pakikisama, 7, 10, 11–12, 15–16, 17–18, 31–32, 42, 47, 49–50, 53, 57, 61, 62, 64, 91, 104–05, 109, 110, 113; definition, 157

palusot, 64; definition, 157
paternalism, 17, 18, 57, 59, 63, 109–10
Patients' Rights Act of 1995, 133–40
patients. *See* Patients' Rights Act of 1995; physicians
personalism, 7, 9–10, 12, 15, 18, 23, 61, 104, 107
Peschke, C. H., 92
pharmaceutical industry 49–50, 108, 119. *See also* drugs; Generics Act
Pharmacists for Life, 130
Philippines, general information and statistics, 151–56
physicians, 47–51, 56–59, 76, 81, 84, 86, 113–16; and patient relationship, 3, 5, 15–18, 24–29, 35, 36–38, 42–43, 63–64, 86, 94–96, 98–99, 104–06, 109; Code of Ethics, 141–50. *See also* paternalism; Patients' Rights Act of 1995
population, control, 30, 32; in Philippines, 155
principlism, vii, xi, 4–5, 8, 15, 18, 70, 107
privacy, patient's right to, 4, 12, 81, 136
prostitution, 83

Relman, A. S., 50
resources. *See* allocation of resources
rhythm method. *See* birth control
Rie, M., 78
Roman Catholic Church. *See* Catholicism
Rosales, V. J. A., 91
Roth, L. H., 48

Schüklenk, V., 81
Second Vatican Council, 54, 125
sexuality, viii, 127
St. Paul, 53–55, 125, 128
Stark, F. H., 49
stealing (from institutions), viii, 61
Steinbrook, R., 84
Sushinsky, A., 81

Todd, J. S., 49
traditional birth assistant (TBA), 104–05. *See also* hilot
truth telling, vii, viii, 15, 62–63, 81, 86, 95–96

utang na loob, 7, 10, 12–13, 15–16, 18, 26, 40, 42, 47, 49–50, 53, 55, 57, 61, 64, 65, 91, 94, 104–05, 107, 113; definition, 157

walang budhi, 53; definition, 157. *See also* budhi
walang hiya, 40; definition, 157. *See also* hiya
walang utang na loob, 12, 65–66; definition, 157. *See also* utang na loob
World Health Organization (WHO), 114–15

Zuger, A., 84